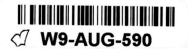

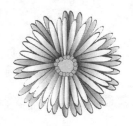

A Daybook for Nurses:
Making a Difference
Each Day

Especially for you,
from a
Sigma Theta Tau International
author.

All the best

S Hudacek

Books of Stories by and about Nurses from the Honor Society of Nursing

A Daybook for Nurses: Making a Difference Each Day, Hudacek, 2004.

Making a Difference: Stories from the Point of Care, Volume 2, Hudacek, 2004.

Pivotal Moments in Nursing: Leaders Who Changed the Path of a Profession, Houser and Player, 2004.

Ordinary People, Extraordinary Lives: The Stories of Nurses, Smeltzer and Vlasses, 2003.

The HeART of Nursing: Expressions of Creative Art in Nursing, Wendler, 2002.

Stories of Family Caregiving: Reconsideration of Theory, Literature, and Life, Poirier and Ayres, 2002.

As We See Ourselves: Jewish Women in Nursing, Benson, 2001.

Cadet Nurse Stories: The Call for and Response of Women During World War II, Perry and Robinson, 2001.

Making a Difference: Stories from the Point of Care, Hudacek, 2000.

The Adventurous Years: Leaders in Action 1973-1999, Henderson, 1998.

For more information and to order these and other books from the Honor Society of Nursing, Sigma Theta Tau International, visit the society's Web site at www.nursingsociety.org/publications, or go to http://www.nursingknowledge.org/stti/books, our catalog page for the Web site of Nursing Knowledge International, the honor society's sales and distribution division, or call 1.888.NKI.4.YOU (U.S. and Canada) or +1.317.634.8171 (Outside U.S. and Canada).

Sarah:
Thank you for your
Contribution to
LRONN 2004

A Daybook for Nurses:
Making a Difference
Each Day

Sharon Hudacek, RN, PhD

Sigma Theta Tau International
Honor Society of Nursing
Indianapolis, Indiana, USA

Sigma Theta Tau International

Publisher: Jeff Burnham
Acquisitions Editor: Fay L. Bower, RN, DNSc, FAAN
Development Editor: Carla Hall
Proofreader: Linda Canter
Composition and interior design by Rebecca Harmon
Cover design by Gary Adair

Printed in the United States of America
Printing and Binding by V.G. Reed & Sons

Sigma Theta Tau International
550 West North Street
Indianapolis, IN 46202

Visit our Web site at www.nursingsociety.org for more information on our books and other publications.

ISBN: 1-930538-13-8

Library of Congress Cataloging-in-Publication Data

Hudacek, Sharon.
  A daybook for nurses : making a difference each day / Sharon Hudacek.
     p. cm.
  Includes bibliographical references and index.
  ISBN 1-930538-13-8 (pbk.)
  1. Nurses--Anecdotes. 2. Nursing--Anecdotes. I. Title.

RT82.H775 2004
610.73'02--dc22
                                                    2004024572

04 05 06 07 / 9 8 7 6 5 4 3 2 1

I would like to dedicate this book to my husband, Stephen L. Hudacek, and my boys, Stephen and Chas. They have given me the gifts of love, wisdom, generosity, and many precious moments in time.

Acknowledgements

The words of nurses inspired me to write this book. The goodness of the words of nurses. Words that are often spoken only by nurses. Words that are often only heard nurse to nurse. These soft words, tender phrases, and spiritual thoughts are now documented. They are our legacy. They are a part of our profession forever.

I wish to thank so many people who have given me constant support and inspiration. Beginning with the wonderful nurses of the Florida Nurses Association—I wish to thank all of you for years of clinical exemplars. Your exemplars represent the very best in nursing care. I cherish your work. Thanks to Dr. Francis Smith, Willa Fuller, and Dr. Patricia Quigley for sharing with me the many talents of your nurse colleagues.

To Dr. A. Elaine Bond and my colleagues at Brigham Young University, College of Nursing, who contributed to the 50th anniversary celebration called *Healers Art;* thank you for sharing your words with me. To Bonnie Wesorick for her writings on nursing leadership. To my research assistants, Mary Bea Maslar and Judith Doherty, for their work in this qualitative project. To Dr. James Pallante for his support in my research endeavors. To Dr. Patricia Harrington and Dr. Donna Carpenter (best buddy) and colleagues in the department of nursing at the University of Scranton. To Alice Lord and Dawn Mazurik—you really came through for me!

To Elizabeth Kuhns Douglas for being a creative force and friend. Thanks Elizabeth for always seeing the coffee cup as half full! I am entirely grateful for your professionalism and support. To my dear Birthday Club friends, Donna, Stacey, Mar, Kath, Gail, Joanne, and Ro. You are always there, through thick and thin. To my sisters Kim and Deb and my mother and father, Kay and Charles Smith. No one could have a better family than the Smith Family.

To Dr. Fay Bower and Jeff Burnham at Sigma Theta Tau International. Thank you for your guidance and encouragement. It is because of you that this daybook was written. You gave me a chance to be creative in 2000. Five years later, you gave me another chance. I tremendously appreciate it.

Finally, to my husband Steve and my sons Stephen and Chas who taught me that the greatest pleasure in life is love!

About the Author

Dr. Sharon Hudacek is an associate professor of nursing and the director of the LPN to BSN program of the University of Scranton. She is the founder of the Making a Difference Foundation, an organization that funds nursing scholarships for LPN students returning for a bachelor's degree in nursing. All *Making a Difference* book profits support this foundation. Her specialty is adult health nursing and pharmacology. She teaches senior nursing students in the three clinical settings at Mercy Hospital Scranton: neuro, orthopedics, and renal, which she considers the most valuable role in her teaching career. The recipient of many honors and awards, she has written *Making a Difference: Stories from the Point of Care*, which won the Best of Book Award in 2003, presented by Sigma Theta Tau International. Dr. Hudacek is married and lives with her husband, Stephen, and their two sons, Stephen and Chas, in Moosic, Pennsylvania. She is homeroom and lunchroom mom and a dedicated volunteer for Scranton Prep and Marian Catholic Schools in Scranton Pa.

Table of Contents

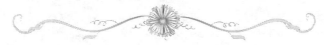

Introduction

Some say that the story has magical powers because it allows us to share a vivid encounter. It helps us describe our work, our family, or the best parts of life. Words and reflections carry meaning. Having reviewed more than 500 nurses' memoirs during the past 10 years, I've learned that nurses speak powerfully and eloquently. Their words are passionate, captivating the mind and igniting the spirit. The nurses' quotes, anecdotes, and observations in this book come from my research in collecting nurses' memoirs from all over the world.

Nurses are incredible storytellers. Did you ever meet a nurse without a great story? Nurses learn, teach, and inform those they are connected to by using stories. They learn about the complexity of caring by using words and stories. The wisdom nurses gain from years of clinical practice is profound. Their words are powerful tools that enlighten our minds. In this book, nurses share personal anecdotes, observations, and seeds of wisdom that inform us. The words do, in fact, soothe our souls.

This book is a daybook—a daily reminder of the greatness of nurses. It illustrates the written and spoken work of nurses in a daily chronological format—in the form of poems, quotes, prayers, or even short narratives. The words within may evoke strong feelings as nurses detail experiences etched in their memories. The thoughtful reader will have access into the very art of nursing and the beauty inherent in this profession. This book honors the great words of nurses. The reader can receive daily inspiration by journeying through its contents each day. Keep this book at your bedside, in your pocket, or at your desk. Keep your own personal notes in the text or at the end of the book. Allow this daybook, written just for nurses, to provide you with the pride and peace you have earned and so richly deserve.

A number of daily entries that appear in this daybook were taken from other books published by Sigma Theta Tau International, including:

Making a Difference: Stories from the Point of Care, Second Edition (2000)

Ordinary People, Extraordinary Lives: The Stories of Nurses (2003)

The Heart of Nursing: Expressions of Creative Art in Nursing (2002)

Pivotal Moments in Nursing: Leaders Who Changed the Path of a Profession (2004)

Cadet Nurse Stories: The Call for and Response of Women During World War II (2000)

As We See Ourselves: Jewish Women in Nursing (2001)

Stories of Family Caregiving: Reconsiderations of Theory, Literature, and Life (2002)

For more information about these and other books published by Sigma Theta Tau International, visit www.nursingsociety.org/publications. If you would like to read more stories by and about nurses, or share your own stories with other nurses, please visit the home page of Nursing Knowledge International, the sales and distribution division of Sigma Theta Tau International, at www.nursingknowledge.org/stti/books.

Thanks for being a nurse and for caring for the world, one person at a time.

January

The cool air rushes in, and the world is quieted by a blanket of dancing snowflakes. A warm fire, the scent of spruce and cinnamon is in the air. January is a time of new beginnings, promises, and crisp change. It's a chance for resolution and tenacity. What will this New Year bring for the extraordinary nurse?

When you do the common things in life in an uncommon way, you will command the attention of the world.

—George Washington Carver

January 1

As a nurse, I must help and share, laugh and suffer with my patients.
A human being is not complete unless he or she can share with others.
Giving of oneself is the greatest gift.

—Marlene Cesar

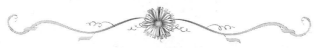

January 2

My personal goal: To improve the quality of life for every patient and family
whose lives I touch. It may involve my nursing assessment skills, or may simply involve holding a hand, stroking a forehead, reading a poem, lighting a
candle, saying a prayer, or just being there at two o'clock in the morning.

—Judy Loeffler

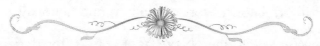

January 3

Respect is not a one-time act but a commitment to a way of being
together as humans.

—Bonnie Wesorick

January 4

Nursing is a science, but it is also about the art of caring.
That is what makes it more than a job!

—Nour O'Quinn

January 5

Tucking You In

I walked by your room today.
I'm not your nurse.
I don't even work on this floor.
But you called out.
"Nurse!" you beckoned, looking at me.
As I walked past your room
I stopped.
I considered whether or not to enter.
I did.
I found a little wisp of an old woman
Lying in bed.
You looked so very vulnerable.
Then, you spoke.
Softly, yet with urgency, you asked,
"Where's Mama?"
I stopped,
Trying to digest your statement.
It wasn't the fact that you were confused,
That was apparent.
But I thought about
How you must have felt.
(Where's Mama?)
Then I tucked you in,
I hugged you
And told you to go to sleep.
That Mama was
Not far away.

—Mary Majkut

January 6

The true heroes in this world are children with cancer. Mariah Carey sings about heroes, and this song reminds me of the unbelievably strong children I have cared for:

And when a hero comes along, with the strength to carry on, when you cast your fears aside, you know you can survive.

And when you feel that hope is gone, look inside you and be strong, And you'll finally see the truth that a hero lies in YOU.

—Maryann Godshall (Mariah Carey "Hero," [from the album Music Box] 1993. Copyright held by The Island Def Jam Music Group/Universal Music.)

January 7

In reflection on my nursing career, I realize my experience in nursing with families has enabled me to grow professionally and personally. I also realize each time I reach out and embrace a family there is tremendous risk for inner pain; yet the richness gleaned from immersing oneself in a nurse-patient relationship can never be replicated.

—Susan Parnell Scholtz

January 8

During a nursing clinic session in a Kurdish community, I fell into conversation with an elderly man who had brought a Russian man of Jewish faith to the clinic to pick up medications. I noted the elderly man had a faded series of numbers tattooed on the inside of his arm, horrifying proof he had been in a Nazi concentration camp. In that same room at that same time there were Baylor students (mostly Baptist), Catholic volunteers, Kurds (mostly Muslim), an Armenian family (history shows that Kurds participated in the attempts to exterminate the Christian Armenians 1894-1915), and a Buddhist caseworker. Moments like this help me remember the beauty and power of this work.

—Charles Kemp

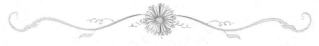

January 9

Even though all I could do in the final stages of her death was to keep her comfortable, I did it with compassion and caring.

—Cathy Bullick

January 10

There is not a shortage of nurses… The real problem is there is a shortage of hospitals where nurses want to work.

—Linda Aiken *(Pivotal Moments in Nursing, p. 226)*

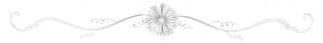

January 11

In all my studying, and as much as I try to become the best nurse, it is impossible to surpass the healing nature of God. He created our bodies, and He makes the rules.

—Stacey Bayles Clark

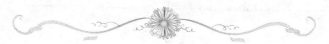

January 12

A nurse chooses whether to care personally about a patient. I chose to care deeply about a boy named Matt—to love him as a son, and he passed away. The pain of separation is the price for choosing to love. The pain will go away, but the love is everlasting.

—Carolyn Sutherland

January 13

As a nurse, a caregiver, and a patient advocate, there is a connection you have to make. I believe that some hesitate to face the reality of the commitment in connecting with patients.

—Deborah Tchorz

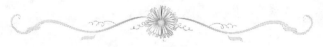

January 14

Bonnie Hunt, also known as the mother of 12 in the film "Cheaper by the Dozen," is beautiful and charming. She is a witty actress with a brilliant mind. What many people do not know is that she has roots deeply set in nursing. For many years in the northwest section of Chicago, Bonnie served as a candy striper and a nurse's aide. She worked as an oncology nurse at Northeastern University Hospital for five years. "You gain a certain maturity from being a nurse in a cancer ward… Call it my extra gift… without it, I would be devastated every day in Hollywood."

—Interview with Barry Koltnow, *Orange County Register*, December 2003

January 15

As I sat with my patient for an hour the night before he went into surgery, I was truly touched. I cared about my patient and his concerns, and by taking the time to listen to him and address some of his concerns, I was able to show I cared. By the time the end of the shift came around, he was not just my patient, he was also my friend. The anxiety and grief he was experiencing were massive, and he needed support. I was the one who had to initiate the relationship, though. That night I learned that creating strong nurse-patient relationships is the first step in establishing trust and unity in care, and providing holistic nursing. It is my responsibility to create it.

—Malesa Weber

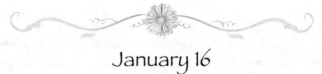

January 16

It is my hope that in my career as a nurse, I will be able to dedicate myself fully to my profession, and know with assurance I have truly been able to make change happen.

—Courtney A. Sudweeks (*The Healers Art*, p. 123)

January 17

Today will always take care of itself, but a leader should always be looking at tomorrow.

—Vernice Ferguson (*Pivotal Moments in Nursing, pg 103*)

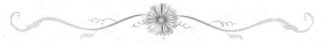

January 18

The spirit of nursing is seen in the ways nurses "are" with patients that is the actions they take as they give of themselves in the caring-healing mission.

—Sharon Hudacek

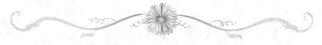

January 19

It was then that I realized that nursing takes place in more areas than just a hospital… it could be in a funeral home, a parking lot, a car, and most of all… in one's heart!

—Francine Zabkar

January 20

Once a patient and the family said they loved me. The love is still here.

—Linda M. Rice

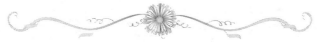

January 21

I will always remember special families for the graciousness they showed me in their time of sorrow and sadness.

—Dana H. Wilson

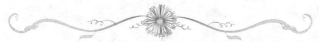

January 22

We may not be able to cure them, but we, through our love and care, can make a difference in the time left.

—Irene Piazza

January 23

I once thought I needed "skills" to be a great nurse. I have learned however, that far more important than what expertise I possess is the time and love I am willing to give away.

—Jeffrey R. Murray

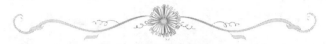

January 24

I left a home visit once profoundly affected. Perhaps it is because of the high degree of trust patients place in us by confiding their deepest concerns.

—Deanna Gordon

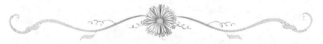

January 25

Nursing is a profession that heals the patient as a whole and not just physically. It is precisely the holistic healing that drew me into this profession

—Allison Ash Malnar (*The Healers Art*, p 30)

January 26

I have chosen to be a nurse. This means I will come in contact with all types of people. I need to give love unrestrained, change my heart, and not allow myself to think judgments against others.

—Ellen S. Baird

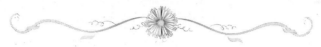

January 27

As nurses, we are taught to be advocates for our patients. However, our judgmental attitudes and prejudices often become an obstacle to patient advocacy.

—Mary Scarbrough

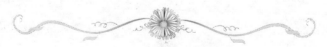

January 28

I learned the skill of crocheting in the summer of 1981. Now I know why my grandmother insisted that it was important. I finished an afghan for a patient named Catherine so she could have peace and move on to the next world.

—Cara Reed

January 29
Heart and Hand

There are forces on the edge,
Forces of light and darkness,
Forces of spirit and heroism, forces of change
That we may welcome or fear.
There are forces that teach us how to live more fully
In the center of our lives.
When I allow myself
To really know about life's little illnesses,
They turn into miracles of recovery.
The sound of my husband's heartbeat
As I lie next to him at night
Becomes a gift of awe and wonder,
And the moment of this discovery
Becomes a moment of pure joy and gratitude.
—Dianne Duchesne

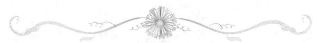

January 30

My patient told me, "Today a baby angel came, and he is sitting on the bottom of my bed. He is my son Jared, whom I lost at three weeks old. He has come to bring me to Heaven with him. So I must say goodbye my friend, and thank you for your loving care." She died that day. Her family was fulfilled by this story, and convinced she was now at peace in heaven.
—JoAnn Slosek

January 31

To be able to be present, to watch and wait, for that moment when a soul makes its journey from this world into the next is a true blessing. To know that you have made a difference for someone and his or her family is an affirmation for why you became a hospice nurse.

—Debra Butcher, on being a hospice nurse

Let no one ever come to you without leaving better and happier.

—Mother Theresa

February

February is a time to dream; a time to love. It is a month for remembering why you chose this nursing profession. Was it love? Not in the quixotic sense of the word, but rather love for humankind. It may be love for the work you do, love for fellow man ... or a combination of both. What in nursing romances you?

Love is like a beautiful flower which I may not touch,
but whose fragrance makes the garden a place of delight just the same.

—Helen Keller

February 1

I remembered the many times that prayer was the only thing that I could do in many situations that seemed helpless.

—Marty Downey

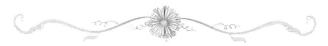

February 2

I have yet to figure out what attracts different people to each other. I have been a nurse for more than 20 years, and I have bonded with some very wonderful patients.

—Debra Woodruff-Caper

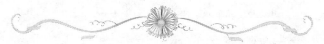

February 3

The way my nonverbal patient was staring at me—the way his eyes followed me wherever I went—led me to believe he recognized my voice. I kept staring back at him, and in his crystal blue eyes, I could see so many things.

—Courtney A. Sudweeks (*The Healers Art*, p. 123)

February 4

An emergency nurse must accept a certain amount of "lack of closure."
After a patient leaves the emergency room setting, often the outcome is
never known.

—Melissa Blevins Jones

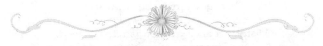

February 5

Several years ago I was called to make a visit to a cancer patient who was
in a lot of pain. No pain medication was available that worked very quickly,
so a call to the physician gave us quick access to concentrated liquid
morphine.

When I entered the home, "Mr. C" was sitting up in a recliner, clutching the
arms and frowning—clearly in much pain. I introduced myself, told him I
was going to give him a dose of the morphine ,and THEN we would talk.
Several minutes after administering the dose he was relaxed; he looked up
at me, and said, "You're beautiful." At that I laughed and said "Gee, I don't
hear that much anymore, not even from my husband." He replied with a
twinkle in his eye, "Give him morphine."

—Nikki Hill

February 6

Cock-a-doodle-doo Angel

It was a pleasure to meet you
The other night, sir.
You see, it had been
A terrible evening in the ER.
One of those low blood sugar,
High bladder level,
"What am I doing here?" nights.
Then, you arrived by ambulance:
88-year-old male, weakness,
History of anemia secondary to GI bleed.
You made your entrance,
All 115 pounds of you
Wrapped up in blankets.
You, with your dark, beady eyes,
Toothless, caved-in mouth
And protruding chin.
Your sparse hair stuck out
Every which way.
You laid in bed sizing me up.
Now, this made me a bit curious.
I wondered how it was
That you had the strength
To look so stern and intent.
You continued to watch me.
You lifted your right hand
Very slowly.
With eyes fixed on me
You touched your left wrist.
You asked, "What time is it?"
But before I could answer,
I heard a very distinct "cock-a-doodle-doo"
From your watch.
Your hard, coal eyes continued to watch me.
Then, you broke out
Into a great big grin
And I discovered you.
My patient was a trickster!
I identified you as such
And you howled with laughter.
I howled with laughter.
My grim evening had suddenly vanished.
Thank you, Angel
With the Cock-a-doodle-doo-watch!

—Mary Majkut

February 7

A patient once said something simple yet profound, "You talk nice to me." I took her hand, looked in her eyes, and responded: "You know what? I like it when people talk nice to me, too." Those few words reminded me of how powerful we are in the lives of the patients in our care.

—Elizabeth L. Santley

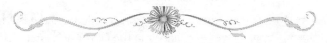

February 8

Get to the table and be a player or someone who doesn't understand nursing will do it for you.

—Loretta C. Ford (*Pivotal Moments in Nursing*, p. 14)

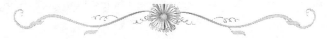

February 9

After emergency surgery, I visited him that evening. Though on a ventilator, he squeezed my hand and gave me a half grin. His wife was appreciative of all we had done.

—Debbie Kennedy

February 10

I am a firm believer that other doors will open when one closes.

—Tyrone Brown

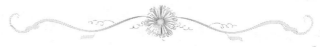

February 11

I'm six-foot-three, male, muscular, African American, and a bald nurse (by choice). Sometimes I see myself in the mirror and I get scared!

—Tyrone Brown

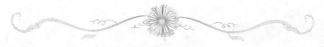

February 12

At times, it can be a frustrating job. You work hard to stabilize and intervene in someone's "crisis" and hope it helps, but never to know for sure if it made a difference.

—Susan Collins

February 13

What is so profound in nursing is the ability and capacity of nurses to open their hearts to the feelings of others, no matter how difficult that may be, at times.

—Sharon Hudacek

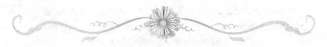

February 14

Valentine's Day was the day I met Joe. I made Joe a valentine, and he insisted I put it up on his TV so it blocked his view of the screen. It made me laugh, but I also felt special because he liked it and such a simple gesture truly meant the world to him.

—Hayley Peterson (*The Healers Art*, p. 112)

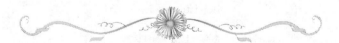

February 15

The sight of someone so sick completely overwhelmed me. I left the room, cried for her, and tried to regain my composure before returning.

—Camille A. Craw (*The Healers Art*, p. 121)

February 16

A Soldier to Honor and Praise

Sometimes it hurts when we love those we help most,
For we face their deaths and heartaches.
Our hearts would grow weary without some great souls,
Who give us more help than they take.

One patient warrior we have helped through the years,
Shares courage and strength when she comes.
She shows us how humor and laughter defend,
Far better than weapons or guns.

She doesn't realize that so many admire
Her courageous and stubborn ways,
That earn her a place with the veterans of war,
A soldier to honor and praise.

Her eyes look much older than her face,
She's aged far beyond her years.
Lines of exhaustion and tiredness,
Compete with lines of good cheer.

This horrible battle is not overseas,
Nor deep in the inner cities,
This endless battle rages all through her mind,
As she struggles for sanity.

There is no real safety, there is no sweet peace,
Watchful enemies have her pinned.
But always she'll have her very best weapon,
She'll fight and she'll laugh 'til the end.

—April C. Johnson

February 17

Humanitarian work has to be one of the most meaningful ways to give of
self and follow the example of the Savior.

—Sandra Mangum

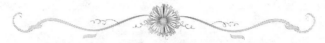

February 18

I felt no one should die alone, so I just sat there with him until he died. I
hope someone will be there for me when I die so I don't die alone.

—John P. Lussier

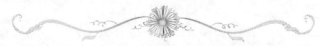

February 19

Handel's "Messiah" was surely not composed in a single day. Nor does a
new nurse master the art of nursing after his or her first shift.

—Lyndsie Oldroyd (*The Healers Art*, p. 130)

February 20

Even in difficult times, there still are great reasons to be a nurse.

—Anonymous

February 21

I know that we do the work of the Samaritan; and I know there is scriptural basis (in all religions) for such work, but it just seems like what we do.

—Charles Kemp

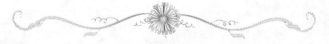

February 22

I received a note from a patient's daughter. She wrote, "I thank you for never being too busy to lend an ear to me. It truly helped me, and I only hope I can return the favor. My dad always felt that you liked and respected him, and he never lost his dignity or hope."

I have that letter still to this day.

—Nina Flanagan

February 23

Without a doubt, advanced medical technologies, medicines, and nursing care bring patients well past their life expectancy.

—Barbara T. Lorenz

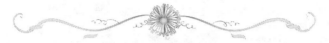

February 24

The next time we are faced with an impossible situation, where a positive outcome seems far from reality, just sit back and "believe."

—Maryann Godshall

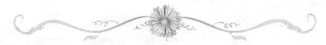

February 25

Each time I see children waiting for our care and look into their beautiful faces, I feel as if I am standing next to the Savior as he calls the children to come for a blessing.

—Sandra Mangum

February 26

Another nurse and I arranged to have a patient admitted to the hospice inpatient unit so her daughter could have a short "respite period." She cried in gratitude and stated, "You're the only people who helped us." It was a good day to be a nurse.

—Name withheld by request

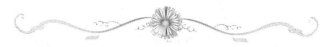

February 27

I began to pray the rosary. This comforting ritual always seems to fill me with a warm glow.

—Marty Downey

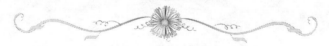

February 28

Like throwing a pebble into still water, I'll never know what the long-term ripple effects will be of the care I give. I'm just a staff nurse, but I'm going to keep trying to do my best and care for my patients even if they aren't easy to care for. I believe the ones who are hardest to love are the ones who need love the most.

—Iris Davis

What does love look like? It has the hands to help others. It has the feet to hasten to the poor and needy.

It has eyes to see misery and want. It has the ears to hear the sighs and sorrows of men.

That is what love looks like.

—Saint Augustine

March

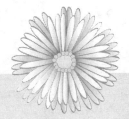

Winter is almost over, and the world is beginning to renew itself with life and growth. The cool breeze will soon be replaced by the scent of grass and seed. Lilacs, daffodils, hyacinth, and crocus bring color and scent to us all. Birds begin to sing. The scent, the sound, the color of spring embraces us, and we are renewed.

To be doing good deeds is man's most glorious task.

—Sophocles

March 1

I want more than anything else to make a difference in the lives of my patients. Even though all of our patients cannot come back and tell us about our caring, my fellow colleagues, the patients, and their families understand the impact of the nurse.

—Linda Rice

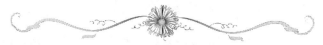

March 2

Two people I have to face each morning and every night: the face in the mirror and God.

—Deborah Tchorz

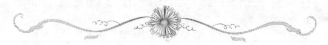

March 3

Working in the OR, nurses often miss out on getting to know their patients. I say a silent prayer for each of my patients as they drift off to that blissful sleep. No matter what their needs are, God, use me as an answer if it's possible.

—Mary E. Scarbrough

March 4

He was learning to read from the books that were stacked next to the IV poles and learning to tell time from the clocks that hung over his chemotherapy equipment. It was an uncertain future for a boy who had barely had time to dream, but who still had large ones.

I began to think about all the things he needed and how little my nursing knowledge and hospital experience mattered to this boy with a potentially fatal disease. There was nothing I had experienced that would compare to the courage this boy was already required to show the world because of the harsh regular treatments he had to endure and the unsure future he looked forward to.

I played checkers with him to pass the time.

I knew the things I had previously relied on to give me the credentials needed to survive nursing heartache and triumph day after day did not include a special insight into hospitalization. I wanted all the patients who were facing the unknown to know that although I had not experienced the many things they were dealing with, I did have something more than under-standing: *I had love.*

—Robyn Carlsen

March 5

Mindprint

I live in a world
Known only to me.
It holds my soul,
My realm of stored truths
That shape my destiny.
—June Heider Bisson

March 6

I have always surrounded myself with the best people to do their jobs,
because I do not want to learn what they already know better than I do.

—Shirley Sears Chater (*Pivotal Moments in Nursing*, p. 36)

March 7

The Old Man

I looked into the eyes of a real old man today
He had yellowing eyes with red streaks
He hadn't spoken an intelligent word in days
But I took time to look
And I saw a young man helplessly trapped in a wrinkled body
A man who silently was screaming for help on the inside
He stayed for a few days
No one ever came to visit him
and then he died.

—Brenda Rushing French (The HeART of Nursing, p. 23)

March 8

I've learned that too often we nurses become task-oriented and feel like we know what is right for the patient. Once patients are given the opportunity to express their feelings and concerns, and to have someone listen, they are able to choose the best path to take for their families.

—Jeffrey Ahsinger

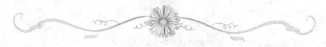

March 9

Creativity and courage help us know how to reach out and help those with particularly unique needs.

—Mary H. Allen

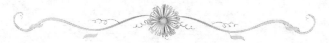

March 10

I have learned that as nurses we can help provide strength with just a word, a touch, or only our presence.

—Cathy A. Yee

March 11

Telling people what they "ought to do" based on our view of the world is not likely to change individual behaviors or significantly impact population health status indices. Life is much more complex.

—Diana P. Hackbarth

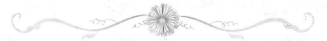

March 12

Nurses are brave and often heroic. Only those who use their hearts and hands to heal and comfort know the true meaning of the work that nurses do. Quiet, peaceful, and satisfied, nurses are the silent workers for humanity.

—Sharon Hudacek

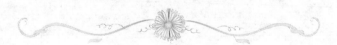

March 13

"One day at a time." These often are words I tell patients and parents, and they are also the core of my care giving. Everyday I have an opportunity to enhance the healing process of my patients by using a holistic approach.

—Sandra Blackington

March 14

Humor has always been important to me because it helps me relax in stressful situations and feel more comfortable in new environments. Humor alleviates stress and allows both nurses and patients to have a diversion. In my own life, humor does so much more than alleviate stress, it helps me remember experiences more vividly, and it helps me teach people more effectively.

—Cody Charlton (*The Healers Art*, p. 23)

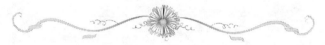

March 15

"I helped her with her hair. Eyebrows penciled, lipstick in place, she absolutely glowed. As I wheeled her into her husband's room, I saw him turn his gaze and attempt a smile. The paralysis slurred his words, I could-n't understand him, but she did. As I rolled her over to him, her hand reached for his and she held it to her face. It was a tearful goodbye; I saw Mr. C. mouth 'I love you,' and she replied the same."

—Lorraine Randall

March 16

Supportive care and effective communication are critical in meeting the health care needs of our patients. Since nurses spend more time than other caregivers with the client during hospitalization, they are in a position to assess patients' psychological and spiritual needs as well as their physical needs.

—Heidi Apsey

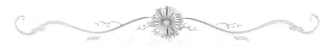

March 17

Slowly we made our way down the dimmed hallways, through the sunporch, and down onto the wheelchair ramp. Soon our bare feet touched the expanse of grass that was the front lawn to the Home. It was 3 a.m. by then, and I was hoping the security guard would not be on his rounds to foil my mission. It was a warm summer night, and phlox were blooming along a stone wall. I guided Horace there to rest and breathe in the delicate fragrance of the flowers. As we sat there, I asked him, "How does the grass feel, Horace?"

"Soft and moist with dew, and oh, so good. I'm almost in heaven," he happily responded.

—Martha Debbie Dixon

March 18

The gifts that patients give me are immeasurable, intangible, colorless, odorless, and neither vegetable, animal nor mineral. The gift of spirit, love, faith, and family. These gifts are wrapped in blessings from God.

—Cara Reed

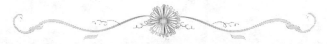

March 19

Everyday, behind the scenes, nurses are, in fact, courageous. They give so much of themselves. Unfortunately, they often don't tell others, but families and patients know. Telling our stories is a way to get the good word out about our profession.

—Sharon Hudacek

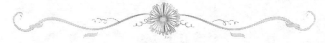

March 20

thought I had to be strong for my patients and families by not showing my emotions. I was wrong.

—Judy Schade

March 21

We purchased a bird named Ethel for our patient Al. She lived in his room, and he kept her on his bedside table. He would stroke her head and allow her to fly around his room. Ethel remained with Al throughout his journey from this life into the next. She sang to him and nurtured him. She was with him until he took his last breath.

—Maryann Rubino

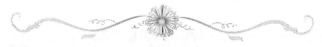

March 22

We learn the basics in nursing school and then with each laboring patient and successive birth, we add a little special something to our memory bank. These nuances allow us to make the difference between an average birth and a fabulous experience for the patient and her family.

—Judith Sorg

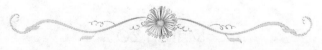

March 23

I realize that *I do love what I do,* and if I can help one person, be it a patient or a family member, then I have done my job well. Often, as nurses, especially in an ICU, we get too involved in the machinery. Nurses need a reality check once in a while, especially in this time of staff cuts and managed care.

—Donna Borer

March 24

Everyone needs to feel loved and cared for so God created nurses.

—Carla Glaus

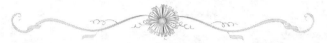

March 25

A patient told me once that I possessed a special gift being a nurse. I never thought of being a nurse as a gift. To me it is what I do for a living. I am just blessed that my job involves giving gifts on a daily basis … love, support, hope, and peace.

—Tina Bears

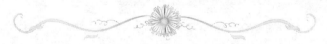

March 26

I noticed my fear today and decided to do something about it. Named it, learned from it, and let it go by going inside for advice from my soul.

—Bonnie Wesorick (*The Way of Respect in the Workplace*, p. 46)

March 27

As a missionary nurse, I had been given the African name Mujinga. The patients I cared for were my "shakena" or namesake. In Africa, I cared for patients by light of kerosene in the absence of electricity. I remember those who passed on. They remain in my heart. Go well my shakena.

—Marjorie Culbertson

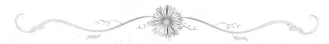

March 28

In the hospital room, human spirit meets human spirit in the hour of greatest need.

—Diane Scheb

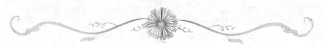

March 29

It's not often that you have as dramatic a chance to help someone or that they thank you for it. More often than not, your efforts are small ones spread over many patients, and you never know which ones were successful.

—Anonymous

March 30

Once I gave a patient flowers to celebrate the end of her chemotherapy.
She thanked me graciously even days later. It was such a simple gesture,
but I realized how much a simple gesture really helps.

—Jennifer Conklin

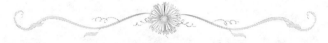

March 31

Nursing is a calling. A profession that can be as great as one wants it to be.

—Deborah Tchorz

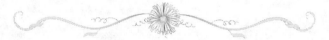

I keep my ideals, because in spite of everything, I still believe that people
are really good at heart.

—Anne Frank

April

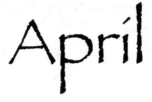

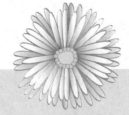

April is beautiful because of the simplicity it brings. Rays of sunlight, the sound of robins, pale blue skies abound. The simplicity of caring for our fellow man motivates nurses. This is caring that is extraordinary, caring that can move mountains.

Kindness in words creates confidence. Kindness in thinking creates profoundness. Kindness in giving creates love.

—Lao-tzu

April 1

The true spirit of caring lives in our hearts and our dreams, and will always live in our memories. It often happens in a single moment, but it changes lives and lifts the soul. It is nursing. It is The Healer's Art.

—Jeffrey R. Murray

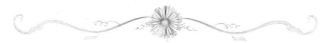

April 2

My favorite thing about caring for patients in the nursing home is hearing about their feelings and their families. Most are at the end of life. I know what it is like to be a friend in end of life care.

—Hayley Peterson (*The Healers Art*, p. 112)

April 3

The first time I held a baby in Labor and Delivery was when I held the still-born. The second time was later that day when I held the live newborn. In just one day, I saw and felt the whole spectrum of the good and bad in Labor and Delivery.

—Tyrone Brown

April 4

Effective pain control involves collaboration between health care providers and patients. Such collaboration helps us practice the art of nursing, as well as the science of nursing.

—Camille A. Craw (*The Healers Art*, p. 121)

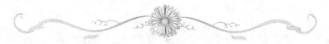

April 5

How arrogant of me to have ever thought that I could understand what is best for the people for whom I care after only spending only a few minutes with them in the ER. I don't know what they have gone through that has shaped them into the person I see laying on a stretcher.

—Iris Davis

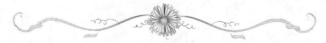

April 6

I feel deep sadness for those who say life is not worth living ... I could not imagine not wanting to see another day.

—Melody A. French

April 7

I had grown during my early days in nursing, from a new nurse with no experience to a nurse beginning to acquire wonderful experiences. My hard work through school and the stress of beginning a new nursing job were well worth the effort.

—Lyndsie Oldroyd (*The Healers Art*, p. 130)

April 8

As long as there is learning, a forward progress, these (mistakes) are growth opportunities, not failures.

—Joyce Clifford (*Pivotal Moments in Nursing*, p. 57)

April 9

How easy it is to judge a person's behavior or appearance; how difficult to put that aside and treat all those we meet with gentleness and compassion.

—Elizabeth L. Santley

April 10

Sweet Mr. Charbonneau

Lying on the stretcher in Trauma Room One.
You lie there so still.
We, in contrast
Are so swift with our motions.
We are so quick and smooth,
You are so still.
We glance at you,
Our eyes imploring.
Respond! Respond!
We hope for resurgence
And you remain still.
We stand at the gate
Between the two planes.
Some of us say, "No! I must have control!"
Others say, "Oh! How the family will cry!"
Yet, others say, "So long."
So long and God bless, Mr. Charbonneau.
You are free to fly above this weathered body,
This plane of familiarity.
It is your time to leave.
And in a brief moment
Undetected by others
My fingers linger with caring intent
Ever so softly on your arm
As I bid you adieu
As you smile upon us
Sweet,
Mr. Charbonneau.

—Mary Majkut

April 11

For me, the children and families I have cared for are not simply faces from the past. There is a place in my heart where I remember each and every one, and I have a unique legacy from each of them that spurs me onward. I am a better nurse because of them. I am a better person because of them.

—Nancy King (*The HeART of Nursing*, p. 98)

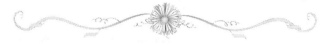

April 12

Nursing and my devotion to God have the same elements, whether it's the passion, caring, or desire.

—Sister Helen Kyllingstad (*Ordinary People, Extraordinary Lives:* p. 3)

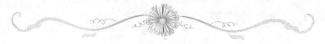

April 13

As nurses, our professional experiences can greatly affect our personal lives, and our personal lives can greatly enhance the care we give.

—Heidi Apsey

April 14

Nurses need to work in coalition with other groups to advocate for social, economic, and environmental changes that afford families the material resources, knowledge base, and community support needed to make healthy, informed choices.

—Diana P. Hackbarth

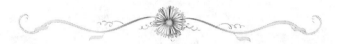

April 15

Grief is a personal issue for both patients and nurses. Not everyone acknowledges loss or handles grief in the same way.

—Mary H. Allen

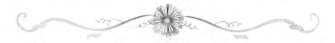

April 16

In the school, home care, hospice, or maybe the emergency room setting, people have been touched by a nurses' healing hands and caring hearts.

—Sharon Hudacek

April 17

My cadet experience challenged me intellectually and physically. I learned about myself and what I was capable of doing. I look back on those years with great nostalgia and with pride that I made it!

—Dorothie Melvin Crowley (*Cadet Nurse Stories*, p. 125)

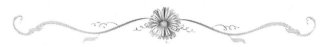

April 18

True nurse angels have similar qualities—their eyes are bright, focused, and compassionate. Their brows furrow as they therapeutically listen, and their mouths curve into smiles of warmth and acceptance. Their voices tell you that they are right there in the moment with you. Their faces are alert, attentive, and ready to respond to the moment.

—Debbie Downey Afasano (*Ordinary People, Extraordinary Lives*, p. 11)

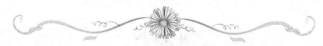

April 19

Often during life-altering experiences, patients and their loved ones need a shoulder to cry on or someone to comfort them. It is important for them to know support is there.

—Lindsey D. Fischer (*The Healers Art*, p. 41)

April 20

I do my job every day to the best of my abilities. As frustrating and hard as it is to jump in and out of people's lives, I enjoy what I do. Every once in a while I can take pride that because of my interventions someone's life was made a little better.

—Susan Collins

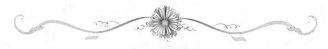

April 21

As a student nurse, and not feeling completely adequate in my knowledge yet, I take comfort in the fact that patients seem to remember the spiritual and emotional needs I meet before they remember what I do for them physically. The holistic approach is what defines the nursing profession.

—Allison Ash Malnar (*The Healers Art*, p. 30)

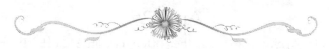

April 22

To be able to be present, to watch and wait, for that moment as a soul makes its journey from this world into the next is a true blessing.

—Debra Butcher

April 23

When I was a little girl, I used to go around with my mother who was considered to be the "neighborhood nurse" … the healer. From her came my desire to be a nurse. I was the first one [in my family] to go into nursing.

—Rose R. (*As We See Ourselves: Jewish Women in Nursing*, p. 94)

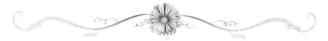

April 24

Nursing care is compassionate, and treating pain is no longer elusive, but a reality.

—Patti Lucarelli

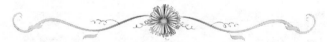

April 25

They endlessly give to so many; they often have little to offer themselves.

—Sharon Hudacek

April 26

The simple thanks you receive from patients' families is the greatest reward one could ever receive for being a nurse.

—Cara Reed

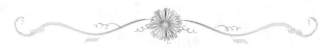

April 27

I must evaluate if I am giving nursing care with a giving heart or a resentful heart. If I can look past the grungy dress or smell and see people as God sees them, then it will be simple to care for them. If my weaknesses were as visible as the smell on my breath and the look of my clothes, then others may not want to be around me.

—Ellen S. Baird

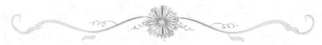

April 28

Because it is deeply ingrained from my nursing education to refrain from giving false hope to patients, I find other ways to communicate that I care, such as listening.

—Heidi Apsey

April 29

Ernest has a full life. He is a nurse, a community leader, and an active member of his church. He is planning to go to law school. He loves being a nurse and may combine, in the future, his nursing skills with law and politics. Whatever the future holds, it is clear, Ernest will continue to make a difference in people's lives…

—Judith S. Mitiguy (*Ordinary People, Extraordinary Lives*, p. 12)

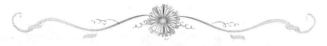

April 30

I may not be able to fix the problems of the world, but I can use the art of nursing to help heal the body and the heart.

—Angie Riches

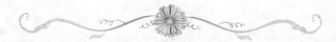

Love doesn't make the world go 'round. Love is what makes the ride worthwhile.

—Franklin P. Jones

May

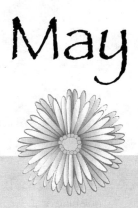

May is about flying; feeling free to impart faith, strength, and tons of courage.

Come to the edge, He said. They said, We are afraid.
Come to the edge, He said. They came. He pushed them, and they flew.
—Guillaume Apollinaire

May 1

Courage, faith, strength, and love—nurses report that these and many more are the gifts they receive from patients and their families.

—Sharon Hudacek

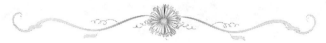

May 2

In this highly technologic time, listening has become somewhat of a vanishing art.

—Catherine Lopes

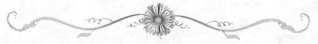

May 3

She wanted to die in front of her window, which looked out onto her lovely garden. We put her bed at the window and she died as she wished, looking out onto the wonderful garden that was so important in her life.

—JoAnn Slosek

May 4

Certain patients teach us to celebrate life, grow in courage, love and commitment. We grow stronger as nurses and more optimistic from knowing them.

—Diana Peirce

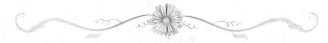

May 5

Hospice nurses know that when patients tell you it is time, it is.

—Sharon Hudacek

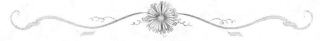

May 6

Knowledge is power and professional practice means a lifetime of commitment to learning.

—Luther Christman (*Pivotal Moments in Nursing*, p. 79)

May 7

Coming closer to her, I could see that with her quaint hands folded as if in prayer, she had quietly left this world.

—Debra Butcher

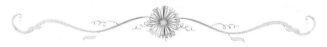

May 8

When I look back now, I realize that while ministering to my patients and families, I was also receiving the benefits of their lives well lived and an example of humanity at its best.

—Michelle C. Steinfeldt

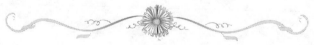

May 9

It's important to call me—even if it's 2 o'clock in the morning—rather than ruminate and worry all night. This is what I tell families who need me.

—Debra N. Fisher

May 10

As nurses we know that our perspective always leaves us with the feeling that more needs to be done and things move too slowly, but the promise is at the end of the verse in Isaiah 58:8, 10. "Then your light shall break forth like the morning, your healing shall spring forth speedily. If you extend your soul to the hungry and satisfy the afflicted soul, then your light shall dawn in the darkness and your darkness shall be as the noonday."

—Penny Phares

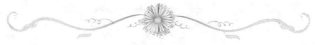

May 11

I learned a lot, and I am grateful for the experience. It gave me a first-hand view of what nursing is all about. Before, I was worried about being able to handle all of the nursing techniques to the best of my ability. However, this is only a fraction of what nursing really encompasses. *Nursing is definitely more than a typical career. Everything nurses perform is important for the nurse's well being, for other health care personnel, and ultimately, for the patient.*

—Erin F. Yamashita

May 12

Nursing Genesis: Our Cross Road

We have come to a crossroad
And we must
Either go or come with you
we linger over the choices
And in the
Darkness of our doubt you lifted the
LAMP of hope and we saw in your
Face the road that
we
should take.

—Mercy Mammah Popoola
(*The HeART of Nursing*, p. 27)

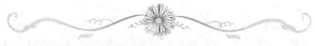

May 13

The family becomes our patient; we nurse the patient and the loved ones.

—Allethaire Cullen

May 14

Our actions had to be swift, each second counted and each intervention was with lifesaving intent.

—Sharon Saunderson Cohen

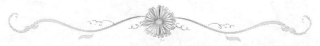

May 15

My nursing career has given me such wonderful satisfaction. I am able to see the benefits of my and my fellow nurses' work daily.

—Gloria H. Denston

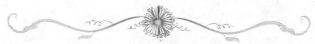

May 16

I learned two things from this military nurse: First, the sacred thing about being a nurse is that we are often with people during their critical life events; second, always listen to the patient.

—Grace Davis (*Cadet Nurse Stories*, p. 178)

May 17

Janet personifies team spirit and encourages camaraderie. But you can't tell Janet that she is someone extraordinary—it's just how she does her job. For Janet, her job and life are always about giving back.

—Geraldine Kelly-Mancuso (*Ordinary People, Extraordinary Lives:*, p. 23)

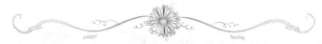

May 18

We are advocates. We assume their role, even if they cannot speak. We are totally responsible for their nursing care—what a truly awesome role.

—Nancy Boyd

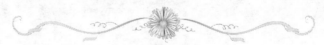

May 19

I was somehow comforted by the fact that at least the last thing this patient saw and heard was a kind face and comforting words.

—Janie Gottschalk

May 20

Taking a few extra minutes, going that extra mile, and giving that added special touch can make a world of difference in a very difficult situation.

—Lisa Lockhart

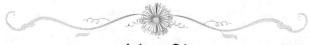

May 21

One day I visited a patient. He asked me if I would give him Holy Communion. This to me was quite an honor. He was a priest. We grew to be great friends.

—Roberta Jerz

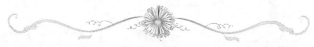

May 22

I put my hand lightly on my patient's shoulder and quietly said, "God bless you. Now you take care of yourself!"

—Iris Davis

May 23

It makes me sad to think that the very simplest of my actions—patience, willingness to listen, respect, kindness—are so foreign to some patients.

—Elizabeth Santley

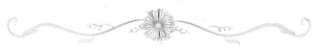

May 24

... At the very least, this man knew we were fighting for his life, his dignity, and his soul. Therefore, we did not fail. We provided a lighthouse in a terrible storm. We continually gave hope when there was none. We gave of ourselves when our own spirits were empty and sad. We all cried tears of empathy and shared in his unabated suffering. And that is why this story had to be told. In that hospital room, human spirit met human spirit in the hour of greatest need.

—Diane Scheb (*Ordinary People, Extraordinary Lives;* p. 175)

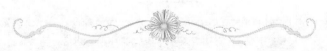

May 25

I have had many experiences in my career that have made me laugh. Many that have made me cry. Some that have made me angry. A few that have made me profoundly sad. But most have made me feel like I made a difference, however small, in someone's life.

—Melody A. French

May 26

Nursing gave me more than nursing skills. Through nursing I learned tolerance, patience, perseverance, and I hope, compassion. Nursing encompassed my entire adult life. Nursing provided me much more than a living. Nursing gave me the self-discipline, self-reliance, the self-confidence to weather the stormy times in life.

—Dorothy Klingla Freeze (*Cadet Nurse Stories*, p. 204)

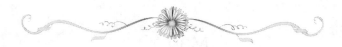

May 27

I have always found great satisfaction in nursing as a career, but my years as a hospice nurse have been the most satisfying of all.

—Thelma Hoogland

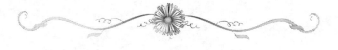

May 28

Heroism. The word symbolizes nursing.

—Sharon Hudacek

May 29

Judaism teaches us to be charitable and compassionate to our fellow man. I cannot imagine choosing another profession over nursing. I find it very rewarding.

—Frieda F. (*As We See Ourselves: Jewish Women in Nursing*, p. 155)

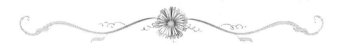

May 30

The good old phrase "you should not get attached to your patients" raced through my mind like a freight train, but I pondered this notion and realized that if one does not get attached, then how does one truly care.

—Deborah Tchorz

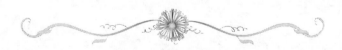

May 31

Nurses who walk the extra mile know they must look harder. They can't settle. They won't settle. Good is not good enough because they want great.

—Sharon Hudacek

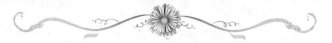

Do not go where the path may lead, go instead where there is no path and leave a trail.

—Ralph Waldo Emerson

June

Lightening bugs, baseball, and lemonade. The front porch beckons you. This is the spirit of June. It's a time for remembering patients—the good times and the bad. It's also a time for remembering the simple kindnesses of nurses and the blanket of caring surrounding so many in need. June is a month of hearing the voice of the patient ... and remembering.

Everybody can be great because anybody can serve ... you only need a heart full of grace.

—Martin Luther King Jr.

June 1

We must try to continue to hear patient voices above the din of the machinery.

—Catherine Lopes

June 2

Patients Whom They Loved

Moonbeams kiss
Nurses miss
Patients whom they loved
Times of joy and those of sorrow
Patients whom they loved

Over the years, many tears for
Patients whom they loved
Critical caring, memories bearing
Patients whom they loved
Smiles and candy
Babies named Mandy
Patients whom they loved
A future of sharing
Big hearts of caring for
Patients whom they loved

—Sharon Hudacek

June 3

I added the small courtesy of picking up coffee for a family member whose husband was very ill. It became part of my morning routine.

—Caryl Wheeler

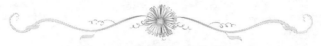

June 4

In nursing, I was taught about the grieving process. Nowhere in nursing school did I get to experience it personally.

—Sharon Saunderson Cohen

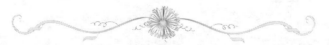

June 5

When the shift starts, you have no idea what care you will need to provide. When a trauma patient arrives, you stabilize, assess, stabilize more, assess more, send the patient off to surgery, deal with psychosocial concerns, get an interpreter for families, save lives, then walk out the door. No one out there can possibly understand the drama behind the work we do. You smile when your significant other asks how your day went, and you answer, "It was just a routine critical care day."

—A. Elaine Bond

June 6

You have to be enthusiastic and passionate about what you do ... and, of course, excellent at what you do and what you believe, so it gets translated to other people.

Vernice Ferguson (*Pivotal Moments in Nursing*, p. 103)

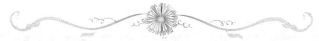

June 7

If you are going to call yourself a professional, then you must call yourself a leader.

—Joyce Clifford (*Pivotal Moments in Nursing*, p. 53)

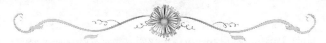

June 8

Much has been written about the healing power of touch. Please do not be afraid of hugging and holding those experiencing a loss and saying, "I am so very sorry this has happened to you." You will offer them more than you realize.

—Mary H. Allen

June 9

As nurses, we know that mistakes have been made because of human error and circumstances beyond our professional control. This is an area that many nurses, daily, remain silent about. They exhaust every mechanism to advocate for the patient. Sometimes it is just too late. Sometimes they are told to mind their own business.

—Sharon Hudacek

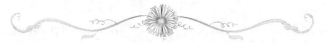

June 10

Each little thing that nurses do for patients, even down to dimming the lights or providing a blanket can touch the heart and soul of a patient.

—Chandra Marie Jeppson

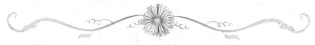

June 11

In the three years I worked with patients in crisis situations, they became my "friends." I knew where and how they lived. I knew where they went for their routine psychiatric care. I remembered what medications they took. I remembered they were people.

—Melody A. French

June 12

Every day I make sure I remember to listen to every patient, for I would never want to miss hearing that last whispered wish.

Catherine Lopes

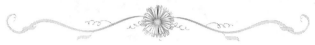

June 13

Cancer gives patients unexpected gifts. Time to smell the flowers, walk on the beach, watch the sunset, look at the moon, and eat whatever they want.

—Connie Shepherd

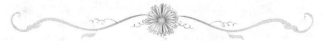

June 14

I continued to visit my patient and teach about nutrition and pain issues. I worried about his anorexia as I watched his gaunt frame lose more weight. Hopefully he would eat some of the soup that I brought him each visit.

—Roberta Jerz

June 15

I found out that the mother of one of our patients only had 30 cents with her. I had four dollars in my pocket for lunch. I collected all the lunch money of the staff, $60. We gave it to this mother.

—Susan Whatley

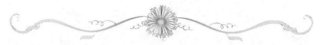

June 16

Pale, fragile looking. Soft, wavy, wheat-colored hair, with furrowing eyebrows atop eyes that scornfully surveyed me. "Well, whatever it is you want, do it and get out of here." I remember thinking to myself, "Oh boy, do I have my work cut out for me today."

—Lorraine Randall

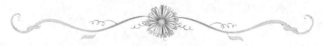

June 17

In a place where so much pain, fear, horror, and loss abounds, would there be some reminders that in the midst of all that, there is love?

—Allethaire Cullen

June 18

You can't imagine how devastating it is for a young, active, and independent woman to be told that she cannot drive because of her history of seizures and potential for more. Suddenly, she was totally dependent on others.

—Sheila Ferrall

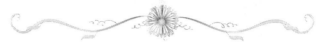

June 19

When I think of my nursing experience in Africa, I think of mangoes. God has given us the mango to put in our stomach when nothing else will grow.

—Nancy L. Fahrenwald

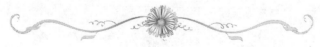

June 20

Emotional pain is expressed by patients in behavior. You can't see the pain, but by certain signs, you can tell.

—Leokadia Bryk

June 21

A mentally handicapped patient I cared for one day sensed that I was upset. He offered me his lemon pie to make me feel better.

—Linda Manley

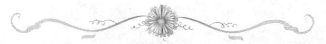

June 22

As a nurse, unequivocally, you value the intangibles.

—Sharon Hudacek

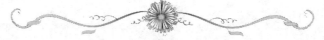

June 23

It is a patient's right to decide what will and will not be done.

—Linda Manley

June 24

Undeniably, nurses are making significant contributions to world health and world peace. They are in military clinics in Iraq, and Guantanamo and helping 9/11 survivors. The face of nursing has drastically changed in the last few years.

—Sharon Hudacek

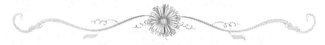

June 25

My inner voice screamed at me. It was so much easier working in a hair salon. The most complicated issue of the day then was "Will this color go with my eyes?" No one was going to die from the wrong choice. Here, in the ICU, there is no control.

—Kathleen Young

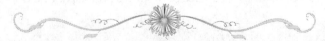

June 26

As a nurse, I learned to appreciate the complexity of the human body.

—Jamison Fleming

June 27

Become aware of actions that leave footprints on the souls, such as for-
giveness, compassion, vulnerability, and trustworthiness.

—Bonnie Wesorick (*The Way of Respect in the Work Place*, P. 42)

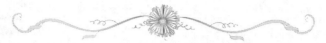

June 28

We were a 14-member volunteer health care team sent to help set up tem-
porary clinics on remote Pacific atolls. These atolls were very primitive, with
no electricity, running water, or industry.

—Victoria Niederhauser

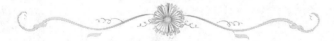

June 29

My pocket is empty but my heart is aching with love and filled with gifts of
beauty … of friendship, hope, dignity, courage, and sacrifice.

—Major Anita Pursino

June 30

Above all, nurses are witnesses to prevailing transformations often beyond our control. Transformations caused by fate, human connections, discipline, and belief in a higher power. All this is done in the spirit of serving others.

—Sharon Hudacek

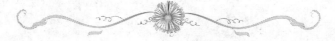

Anything that is of value in life only multiplies when it is given.

—Deepak Chopra

July

July is a month of caring for the soul. The summer is time for *time*. It's time for catching up with old friends. It's time well spent walking on the beach, in the woods, along main street in Small Town, Anywhere. It's about smelling salt water, and pines, listening to the bees buzz, tasting taffy. It's about the contradiction of the coolness of the mountains after the heat of the plains. It's about enjoying the vision of the peaked ocean dunes and the stand of corn along a dusty back-country road. Stand at the water's edge or wherever you find yourself, and nourish your inner being.

If you have nothing at all to create, then perhaps you create yourself.

—Carl Jung

July 1

We can be proud of our skills, our competence, and our compassion. That is what makes the difference between merely going through the motion of caring for a patient, and making things right with their world. That is what makes us nurses.

—Susan Whatley

July 2

Above and beyond the intensive stress, which characterizes every single nursing moment, what is unknown and incomprehensible to many is the heroism of the nurse's heart, which day by day, night by night, creates the unique meanings of nursing.

—Dr. Vassiliki Lanara (*Heroism as a Nursing Value*, 1981)

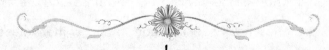

July 3

A simple gesture of just being there can make a difference.

—Jennifer Conklin

July 4

Nurses recognize that their dedicated efforts of caring are not only a mark of excellence, but result in a true gift of love.

—Sharon Hudacek

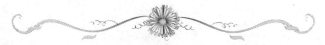

July 5

Many nurses must face the fact that there is little they or others can do to prolong the life of a patient.

—Patricia Benner (*From Novice to Expert*, p. 55)

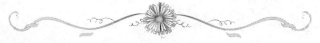

July 6

Minimize the distractions and maximize the tenderness.

—Madeleine Myers

July 7

You don't want to oppose the vision of others. Instead, you should utilize the group vision to obtain motivation through collaboration.

—Ada Sue Hinshaw (*Pivotal Moments in Nursing*, p. 106)

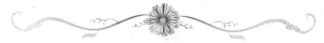

July 8

Reflecting on my nursing experience helps me today to put difficult situations in perspective.

—June Kasiak-Gambla

July 9

We must never lose sight of how critical it is to preserve what makes each of us a nurse.

—Kim Doherty

July 10

Having empathy and love are absolute qualities nurses need to possess
when working in the ICU.

—Chandra Marie Jeppson

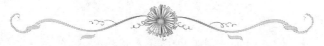

July 11

When working as a staff public health nurse, I received a referral from a
pediatrician who had found elevated lead levels in a Hmong infant whose
family did not speak English. Over the next month, I worked with various
state and local agencies to have the soil surrounding the house tested and
obtain blood samples from all family members for testing for lead levels. All
family members had markedly elevated blood lead levels. The soil around
the house contained high levels of lead and other heavy metals. In
essence, I was able to prevent further occurrences of lead poisoning in
that family and to prevent anyone else from living in a house and environment that contained heavy metals.

—Gwendolyn F. Foss

July 12

"I love you," I whispered. He smiled and squeezed my hand as he lay dying and attempted to whisper, "I love you, too." He died very peacefully the next day. I could not stop the tears. I left with a heavy heart. The next month I received a surprise. It was his rosary beads. I will always cherish that gift.

—Roberta Jerz

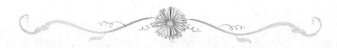

July 13

I think one of the hardest things to cope with effectively in nursing is being the target of misplaced anger.

—Lorraine Randall

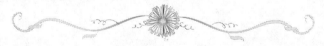

July 14

It was not until the funeral that I realized that it was also my patient's family whom I had cared for over the preceding months, and in turn, I had received equal measure of care and support from them.

—Caryl Wheeler

July 15

Sometimes nurses must also acknowledge the limits of their own understanding.

—Patricia Benner (*From Novice to Expert*, p. 87)

July 16

Welcome

Though you fear this abyss,
where darkness appears endless
first entry feels like falling
and the chill takes your breath,
once you let go
you will arrive at a separate place
where everything, everything matters.

The grief space,
where healing begins,
seems close, intimate,
yet open to a soft wind
from purple hills beyond a broad plain,
scented lightly
with asphodel.

Mark H. Clarke (*The HeART of Nursing*, p. 27)

July 17

I studied and read and learned; it was a degree in nursing I yearned.

—Jennifer McElligott Carley

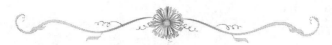

July 18

Relating to others and behaving as a competent professional is the cornerstone of acquiring power resulting from a combination of empathy and a positive personality integrated with intellectual and cognitive skills. Most nurses do possess these attributes.

—Judith Farash McCurdy (*Socialization, Sexism, and Stereotyping*, p. 365)

July 19

Nursing's service is, and always has been, to society.

—Sharon Hudacek

July 20

It is so hard to try to communicate solace to a patient, trying to share soothing words that could ease some pain.

—Leokadia Bryk

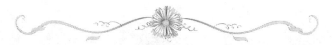

July 21

Ignorance can be effectively decreased through reading, studying, and sharing our knowledge and experiences with other nurses.

—Mariann C. Lovell (*Socialization, Sexism and Stereotyping*, p. 220)

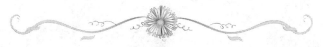

July 22

Frankly, I jumped at the opportunity to become a cadet nurse because it was free, and if I completed the course I could earn more money than I currently made as a clerk. This decision of convenience turned out to be a decision "made in heaven." I loved nursing.

—Florence Blake Ford (*Cadet Nurse Stories*, p. 29)

July 23

I sat there for a while pondering the events of the evening. A young, active woman had walked into an emergency department for leg pain only to find that she had a brain tumor.

—Kathleen Young

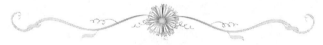

July 24

Each nursing experience I have helps me grow as a nurse, and I integrate each of those experiences into my practice.

—Kathleen Young

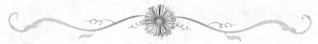

July 25

What a blessing nurses have in caring for the most sick, those patients who need a caring person to love them and give them the support they richly deserve.

—Chandra Marie Jeppson

July 26

From the time I was a small child, I wanted to be a nurse. Back then one had to be a nurse to be an airline stewardess, and that was what I wanted to be. My parents encouraged me in whatever I wanted to do, as long as I had an education or trade after high school.

—Adele A. (*As We See Ourselves: Jewish Women in Nursing*, p. 100)

July 27

As nurses, we are often faced with situations that may puzzle or confuse us. We may not question an action or decision at the moment that it is made, but in retrospect, we may ask ourselves, "Did I do the right thing?"

—Victoria P. Niederhauser

July 28

Nursing requires brains and skill.

—Janet Muff (*Socialization, Sexism, and Stereotyping*, p. 240)

July 29

The terrorists attacked us and planted the perception of fear and terror among us. Like many others, I am more resolved and determined.

Major Anita Pursino, Operation Enduring Freedom

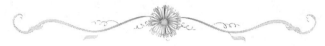

July 30

I loved that I had the opportunity to help ease his great pain, if only for a day.

—Rachel Contreras-Spencer

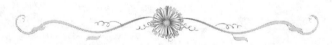

July 31

No one out there can possibly understand the drama behind the work we do.

—A. Elaine Bond

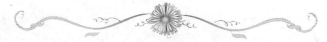

If you find it in your heart to care for someone else, you will have succeeded.

—Maya Angelou

August

August is about touch. The August days warm us like a caress. The words and images of nurses, the powerful statements they make, inspire us each and every day. In this month, nurses focus on the importance of documenting the work of nurses—not only the skill-oriented care, but also the supportive, personal touch that augments nursing care. It's a time to remember to put your stories to pen. To learn from them and pass them along to those who need them.

August creates as she slumbers, replete and satisfied.
—Joseph Wood Krutch

August 1

I have learned that it is not so much what I do that is important, but it is how I do it.

—Ellen S. Baird

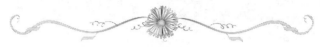

August 2

Our stories afford nursing scholars a special access to the human experience of time, order, and change, and it obligates us to listen to the human impulse to tell tales.

—Margarete Sandelowski (*Telling Stories: Narrative Approaches in Qualitative Research*, p. 165)

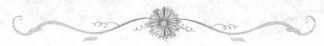

August 3

It occurs to me that nurses do not save their stories, not because they don't value them, but because they don't know that others value them.

—Sara E. Abrams (*Saving Our Stories*, p. 77)

August 4

On the art of nursing: Beauty is not strictly meant to be that which
is beautiful but rather that which takes a form that is satisfying and
appealing to others.

—Susan B. Leight (*Starry Night: Using Story to Inform Aesthetic Knowing in
Women's Health Nursing*, p. 110)

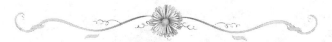

August 5

During the most distressed times, we urgently need stories (nursing)
that illustrate the best of our practice.

—Patricia Benner (*The Wisdom of Our Practice*, p. 105)

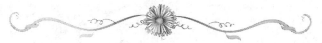

August 6

Caring practices and astute nursing judgment are called "arts" because
they are not predictable or perfect.

—Patricia Benner (*The Wisdom of Our Practice*, p. 105)

August 7

As professionals, we are struggling to develop a theory of nursing ethics without really listening to what our experiences with patients tell us.

—Randy Spreen Parker (*Nurses' Stories: The Search for a Relational Ethic of Care*, p. 34)

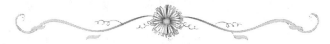

August 8

I cried that day, learning the pain that comes when there are no answers for what has happened.

—Angie Riches

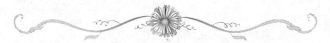

August 9

A nurse's bedside manner impacts a patient's recovery and healing experience. Choosing to make nursing an art is increasingly more challenging and easy to overlook as demands on nurses increase.

—Katie Johnson

August 10

I went over, picked him up, and cradled him in my arms. I bathed him,
clothed him, and held him.

—Rachel Contreras-Spencer (*The Healers Art*, p. 13)

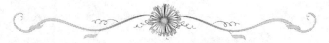

August 11

For attractive lips, speak words of kindness.

—Audrey Hepburn

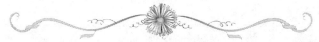

August 12

Nursing skills and knowledge are vital to make a nurse, but compassion and
caring are vital to make a great nurse!

—Marianne Stewart

August 13

Humor alleviates stress and allows both nurses and patients to have a more enjoyable experience.

—Cody Charlton (*The Healers Art*, p. 23)

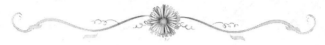

August 14

I am a firm believer in mentors and the strength that relationship can offer another individual.

—Faye G. Abdellah (*Pivotal Moments in Nursing*, p. 139)

August 15

A cloth across a forehead: It couldn't be simpler. Yet that simple act connotes comfort, caring, and human bonding.

—Jeffrey R. Murray

August 16

The Voice of Courage

From the deepest depths it comes,
a voice.
At times it bubbles up
slowly, meekly
calling to be heard
begging attention.
At times it rushes out forcefully
a screaming outcry,
compelling action.
A powerful voice in
Meekness or might.
Could it be the voice of the soul ...
Offering direction,
Purpose, possibilities,
Self,
Offering freedom?
Listen to the voice.

—Laurie Shiparski (The HeART of Nursing, p. 28)

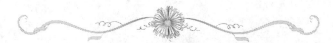

August 17

Sister Helen talks to patients about their treatments in simple words they understand. Both doctors and patients admire her endless patience and teaching abilities. Sister Helen believes all her nursing experiences have led her to this niche, her niche of providing hands-on care. Hands-on care is what Helen loves and intends to do as long as she can.

—Sister Mary Stephen Brueggeman (*Ordinary People, Extraordinary Lives*, p. 25)

August 18

I am solemnly aware of the obligations I assume toward my country and my chosen profession; I shall follow faithfully the instructions and guidance of my instructors and the physicians with whom I shall work; I shall keep my body strong and my mind alert, and my heart steadfast; I shall be kind, tolerant, and understanding. Above all, I will dedicate myself now and forever to the triumph of life over death. As a cadet nurse, I pledge to my country my service in essential nursing for the duration of the war.

—Cadet Nurse Pledge (*Cadet Nurse Stories*, pp. 57-58)

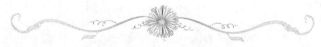

August 19

My patient wanted a song. We picked the song "I Need Thee Every Hour," and we stood at the end of the bed and sang him this song.

—Angela Williams (*The Healers Art*, p. 17)

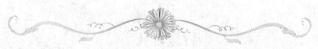

August 20

Apprehension, uncertainty, waiting, expectation, fear of surprise, do a patient more harm than any exertion

—Florence Nightingale

August 21

Nurse work is courageous yet very private. For too many years, nurse work has been silently dismissed like pennies in the fountain.

—Sharon Hudacek

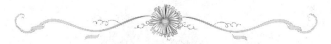

August 22

I never wanted anything but nursing; it has been a perfect career for me. I can make a living, and I feel I'm of help to someone else. At least once every day I've helped someone.

—Gloria G. (*As We See Ourselves: Jewish Women in Nursing*, p. 153)

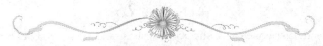

August 23

Nurses and patients are interconnected. Become a part of the healing environment and create harmony.

—Madeleine Myers

August 24

Everyone has a soul and deserves and needs to be loved and cared for.

—Linda Manley

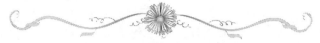

August 25

My religion is very simple. My religion is kindness.

—The Dalai Lama

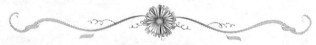

August 26

My job is to dispense care, support families, and do all that I can to send new babies out into the world in the best possible shape, and never underestimate the power of love.

—Kathey Milligan

August 27

The touch of a nurse's hand is as precious as gold.

—Jennifer McElligott Carley

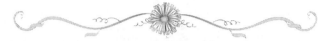

August 28

Nurses know what a big difference a simple gesture can make, such as holding a hand, rubbing a back, or discussing in simple terms what procedure will occur.

—Sharon Hudacek

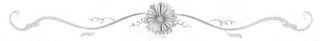

August 29

In providing attention to patient and family alike, we not only care for the emotional well-being of our patients, we in turn receive emotional support from the community of family and visitors. The impact of this is to multiply our value and effectiveness as caregivers and increase our job satisfaction exponentially.

—Caryl Wheeler

August 30

Nurses know the magic of a smile, hug, or nod of approval.

—Sharon Hudacek

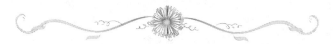

August 31

The technology of neonatal care has dramatically increased survival.
Nurses can lead the health care team in the integration of individualized,
developmentally supportive, family-centered care.

—Sandra Blackington

Stories are medicine.

—Clarissa Pinkola Estes

September

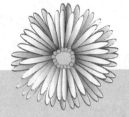

The clarity that September brings is rich. New harvest, clear moon, and maybe a faint chill is in the air. September is the time to gather what is comforting. Family, friends, apple pie, macaroni ... the comfort foods of home. Light a candle, breathe in the scent of cider, enjoy the fact that September is upon us.

Up from the meadows rich with corn, clear in the cool September morn.
—John Greenleaf Whittier

September 1

I witnessed a patient, a farmer, with advanced bowel cancer return home. He only had a few weeks to live. As I traveled down a winding mountain road, I could see him in the distance, a tall, thin, and frail figure carefully rolling an IV pole beside him, admiring his corn stalks as they stood as tall as he. Nothing so wonderful could have hit my eyes and heart. Home to the harvest and home to his favorite possession.

—Cathy Champi

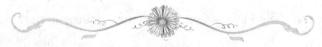

September 2

One day, I baked a fresh apple pie for my patient, Dr. T. Even though it was not on his diet plan, he shared with me that the pie was better for him than any medicine he could ever have taken.

—Dottie Coleman

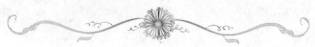

September 3

We have not taken time to look back on the lives we have touched. Rarely, nurses seek credit for their work.

—Sharon Hudacek

September 4

Responsiveness within the context of the nurse-patient relationship means a willingness to accept a patient's invitation to be a close traveling companion on an uncertain journey.

—Randy Spreen Parker (*Nurses Stories: The Search for a Relational Ethic of Care*, p. 37)

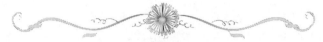

September 5

Saving our stories continues the legacy for those who succeed us in nursing.

—Sara E. Abrams (*Saving Our Stories*, p. 78)

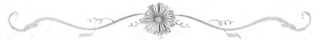

September 6

I continued to rub the back and neck of this 15-year-old girl with cancer. She was shaking uncontrollably and crying. I was thankful she wasn't facing me because the tears were streaming down my face. Soon she fell asleep.

—Jennifer Conklin

September 7

Once I stopped the resuscitation efforts on a patient in order to support the wishes of the family. I have never forgotten the meaning of that event and the effect it had on my current practice. I realize there are many ways to care and to do what is best for the patient.

—Monica Joyce

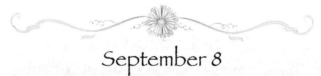

September 8

In death, I have seen six lives saved with organ donations from a young boy. One heart, one set of lungs, one liver, one pancreas, and two kidneys.

—Sylvia Metzler

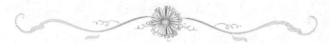

September 9

We are still learning the vocabulary, but with each story a nurse tells, the language becomes clearer.

—Randy Spreen Parker (*Nurses Stories: The Search for a Relational Ethic of Care*, p. 39)

September 10

She lived on a farm all of her life. The last day we moved her to the window overlooking the farm. She was playing her favorite music softly. The curtains billowed with fresh air, and the cows could be heard ever so faintly in the pasture. She passes away gently during the visit, it was a wonderful experience.

—JoAnn Slosek

September 11

By 10:00 a.m., our wold was completely transformed. We were stunned, shocked, angry, and grief-stricken. Our lives would never be the same. But we are nurses, and we did what nurses do. We prioritized, improvised, and mobilized and went where we were needed.

—Melissa Offenhartz (*Nurses Remember 9/11*)

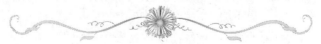

September 12

The development of ideas requires being willing to disseminate the finding and be open to discussion and critique. Critique is a powerful and essential tool to improve the product by putting it out to the brightest minds to evaluate its merit from their unique experience and knowledge base.

—Sue Donaldson (*Pivotal Moments in Nursing*, p. 167)

September 13

Automatic

With a sigh,
The negative pressure unit
Vacuums oxygen
To its sticky sacs,
Exchanging it for carbon dioxide
At the finely regulated capillary membranes
The CO2 dissolves warmly
In the winter air
From the now laughing mouth
Of the child.

Julie Ann Fitch (The HeART of Nursing, p. 51)

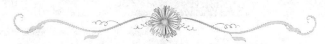

September 14

Nursing offers in my professional life what I can be in my personal life; I look around and see homelessness, unwanted children, lack of access to health care, and nursing [at this Jewish hospital] addresses all of these things, takes care of all these problems.

—Bonnie B. (As We See Ourselves: Jewish Women in Nursing, p. 153)

September 15

Their work is spiritual. God-given, they are the unsung heroes every day.

—Sharon Hudacek

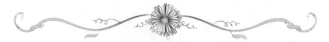

September 16

Know you'll make mistakes; take advantage of the lesson. Know you will make errors; forgive yourself. Know you'll seem unkind and insensitive; recall being loved or loving someone. Know you will meet fear; expose it. Know you will die; prepare by living each moment of this journey.

—Bonnie Wesorick (*The Way of Authenticity in the Work Place*, p. 29)

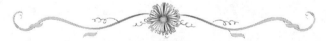

September 17

It was the same thing I felt every time I saw a child born; it was heaven.

—Angie Riches

September 18

We treated her wounds (psychological) and accepted her where she was, and we did our very best to be her door back to normal.

—Nour O'Quinn

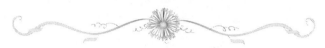

September 19

Every time I tell someone I am a nurse who works with cancer patients, the first response is, "Oh, that must be so sad." Being an oncology nurse can be sad, but it is very rewarding and a privilege. The greatest gift given to me is how to really appreciate life. "If it's chocolate cake you want for breakfast, then chocolate cake is what you shall have.

—Michelle Williams (*Ordinary People, Extraordinary Lives*, p. 191)

September 20

In caring for children, mothers are often the heroes because they advocate so strongly for their children. As nurses, we put the pieces together and send them on the path to discovery.

—Name withheld by request

September 21

Working as a school nurse for a low-income preschool program is an experience different from any type of nursing I've ever done. It is prevention, teaching, and screenings. As a nurse, you really make a great difference in the care of children.

—Name withheld by request

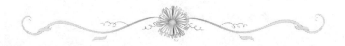

September 22

Organization is the power of the day; without it, nothing is accomplished.

—Sophia Palmer

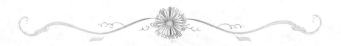

September 23

I once arranged for a patient's dog to be brought to the hospital. I cleared this with the infectious disease nurse and the doctor. He was a beautiful dog, and we were all in tears at the reunion, which happened to be the final day in the patient's life. I made the best decision I ever have made.

—Name withheld by request

September 24

I was in Guantanamo Bay and observed surely the presence of God on earth. We held a religious service in this camp in Cuba. It was a service for healing. The sound of the children singing there ... brought tears to everyone in attendance.

—Kathryn Gaylord

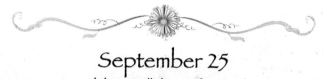

September 25

Administrative responsibilities pull the professional nurse away from the bedside.

—Olivia Miner (*The Healers Art*, p. 70)

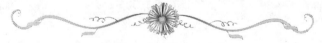

September 26

Once in a while, everyone has one of those incredible experiences, where one learns there is more to nursing than just the application of secular knowledge.

—Rachel Contreras-Spencer (*The Healers Art*, p. 13).

September 27

Health promotion must be a collaborative effort between schoolteachers, nurses, governments, companies, and families. By involving people from a variety of disciplines, health promotion is reinforced and change is more likely.

—Christy M. Spaulding

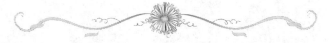

September 28

By taking care of the happiness of other people, we are finding our own.

—Jana Bartkova

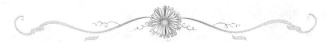

September 29

In Japan, we arranged for one of our patients to use a word processor to make beautiful cards. Her life became rich. It was the best joy for the nurses to see.

—Tomomi Kameoka

September 30

For today, I see the eyes of my patient, and I do not forget him.

—Alzebeta Hanzilikova

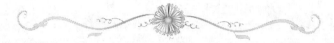

When we truly care for ourselves, it becomes possible to care far more profoundly about other people.

The more alert and sensitive we are to our own needs, the more loving and generous we can be toward others.

—Eda LeShan

October

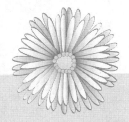

Imagine the work of nurses, gently providing care to heal the body and the soul. See nurses respecting the value of individual patients; see nurses honoring needs and wishes; see nurses offering care, advocacy, and comfort. October is the month for simplicity and comfort. It is a time to prepare for the oncoming chill; the oncoming winter. It is a time for quilts and fires for snuggling. It is a time to take stock of our assets—our harvest of memories and stories. It is a time to relish in the warmth of an unexpectedly warm afternoon, and it is a time to curl up with a good book and a good story. It's a time to tell your stories to your children, your grandchildren, while sitting quietly in a rocking chair or beside a crackling fire. Remember the stories. Always remember the stories.

October is crisp days and cool nights, a time to curl up around the
dancing fire and sink into a good book.

—John Sinor

October 1

What greater job is there than to gently touch and sometimes help heal the body and soul of a kindred spirit?

—Carol Jackson (*The Healers Art*, p. 47)

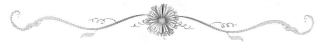

October 2

I remind myself to focus on what I have that is good and right in my life, which always begins the momentum needed to move me ahead.

—June Kasiak-Gambla

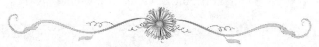

October 3

We concluded that we could not do what nurses do for patients—we could not touch him (it hurt too much), we could not feed him (by the end he could not swallow), we could not tell him that everything was going to be OK (because we knew in our hearts that it was not going to be).

—Diane Scheb

October 4

Each individual has a need for custom care.

—Holly Harwood (*The Healers Art*, p. 50)

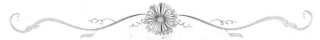

October 5

Bound by paperwork, short on hands, sleep, and energy ... nurses are rarely short on caring.

—Sharon Hudacek

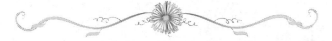

October 6

She had cancer, my nurse friend. She was dying. She cried, and I held her.

—Connie Shepherd

October 7

From now on, I will try to look at the situation from the patient's viewpoint, and not let *my* values get in the way.

—Francine Zabkar

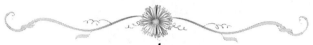

October 8

Expert (nursing) practice embodies the notion of excellence; by studying it, we uncover new knowledge. Thus, theory shapes practice, and practice shapes theory. In the best of worlds, practice and theory set up a dialogue that creates new possibilities.

—Patricia Benner & Judith Wrubel (*The Primacy of Caring*, p. 21)

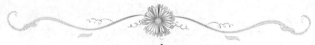

October 9

Being a nurse since 1974 makes it a lot of years in nursing. This "old dog" has seen a lot of changes and advances in medicine. But we all go back to the essential basic skills we first learned in nursing: assessment, communication, and perseverance.

—Penny Kochanowski

October 10

Advocacy means to inform the patient of his or her rights and then support those rights.

—Jennifer Benson

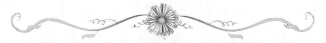

October 11

Build an area of expertise and others will seek you out.

—Margretta "Gretta" Madden Styles (*Pivotal Moments in Nursing*, p. 169)

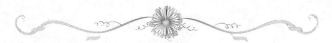

October 12

I handed her a toothbrush, helped her brush her hair, straightened her pillow and linens, handed her a cool washcloth, and got her a snack. If she could feel good about herself, then she could focus on the healing of her body.

—Carolina Jensen (*The Healers Art*, p. 36)

October 13

The day was extremely busy and I was tired. I wanted to just take a break, sit down, and rest my weary feet. Somehow I received the strength and capacities that day that I needed.

—Carolina Jensen (*The Healers Art*, p. 36)

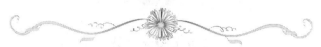

October 14

I walked into the softly lit room and approached my patient, laying my hand on his shoulder. He turned his head and looked up to me. He didn't need to speak. I could read the sadness in his tearful eyes. I leaned down and we hugged for what seemed like an hour, but was only moments.

—Francine Zabkar

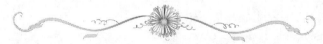

October 15

To provide quality patient care, a nurse must create the opportunity to understand human diversity.

—Holly Harwood (*The Healers Art*, p. 50)

October 16

In recovery from surgery, he reached out his hand to hold mine ... I sat in
the chair at his side watching over him.

—Jennifer Allen

October 17

Past the Signs (In memory of Joel Tower)

I watch your chest move up and down
But it is not our own.
Your eyes are fixed with no response,
Your limbs but stiffened bone.
Your pulse is rapid, your pressure low
And ICP beyond belief.
I wish the nurse in me would go,
Would ignorance bring relief?
My stomach is tied all in knots
But you seem to rest in peace,
Past the signs that are telling me,
You'll soon crash, you, my brother, I see.

—Julie R. Tower (The HeART of Nursing, p. 77)

October 18

We knew that we were fighting for his life, his dignity, and his soul.
We provided a lighthouse in a terrible storm.

—Diane Scheb

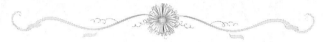

October 19

I sponged his head with cool water, washed his face, and dampened his
hair. His eyes rolled back as he enjoyed the cooling sensation of the
water. I realized he was only a few years older than I was and would be
paralyzed for the rest of his life.

—Maile Wilson (*The Healers Art*, p. 45)

October 20

Participating in any aspect of healing is a humbling, awe-inspiring experience.

—Carol Jackson (*The Healers Art*, p. 47)

October 21

Childbirth is such a miraculous, spiritual event that as a nurse, I just wanted to be part of it.

—Lindsey D. Fischer (*The Healers Art*, p. 41)

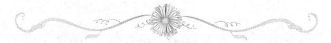

October 22

More than any other helping professionals, nurses attend to the relationship between illness and disease.

—Patricia Benner & Judith Wrubel (*The Primacy of Caring*, p. 21)

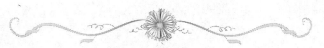

October 23

We focus on the importance of accepting people for who they are, and to respect their differences ... whether they are cultural, religious, or behavioral in nature.

—Holly Harwood (*The Healers Art*, p. 50)

October 24

The feelings, the attachment, the giving by the nurse are … extraordinary.

—Sharon Hudacek

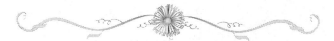

October 25

I tell the story of a man at a gym to whom I had given CPR. He ultimately had angioplasty, and he did well. I was glad I was a nurse that day. I was glad that my CPR technique had been honed to perfection from years of teaching. Then and now I felt both humbled and empowered.

—Joan D. Kramer

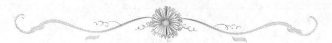

October 26

By offering a hand to hold, whispering honest words of encouragement, and sitting by the bedside, you are able to show support for patients in need.

—Jacy D. Elm

October 27

I am a nurse and am Jewish. The two have been very interrelated in my life.

—Maxine M. (*As We See Ourselves: Jewish Women in Nursing,* p. 155)

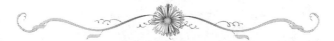

October 28

We can't judge, and we can't take away hope. There is so much we do not know.

—Frances R. Vlasses (*Ordinary People, Extraordinary Lives,* p. 47)

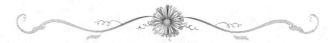

October 29

Parish nursing has provided Michelle with the opportunity to examine her own outlook on life, family, community, and nursing. ... Health ministry and parish nursing have empowered Michelle to bring her faith to nursing, to the community in which she lives and serves, and to her own family.

—Mary Ann McDermott (*Ordinary People, Extraordinary Lives,* p. 27)

October 30

As a nurse, I want my patients to feel they are getting the care they need and deserve.

—Angela K. Leach (*The Healers Art*, p. 64)

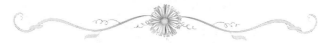

October 31

The Lord is the source of my service as a nurse, and His power enables me to perform miracles in nursing His children.

—Jennifer W. Allen

There are only two ways to live your life. One is as though nothing is a miracle. The other is as though everything is a miracle.

—Albert Einstein

November

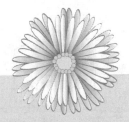

November is the month for thankfulness. Giving thanks for the ability to think and make good decisions. Being thankful for the privilege to work with patients and their families. Appreciating the abundant gifts and talents inherent in this profession.

A thankful heart is not only the greatest virtue, but the parent of all the other virtues.

—Cicero

November 1

Nursing is made or produced by nurses. It is a service, a mode of helping human beings, and not a tangible commodity.

—Dorthea Orem (*Nursing: Concepts of Practice*)

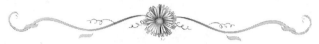

November 2

I was overcome with the incredible sense of grace this man possessed, taking time from his suffering to thank me for what I did.

—Katherine (Katie) Koehn (*Ordinary People, Extraordinary Lives*, p. 163)

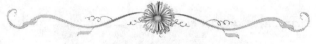

November 3

We never know when as everyday individuals we will have to take on our nurse's role.

—William T. Campbell

November 4

Our time was brief but touching. His recovery was nothing short of a miracle.

—Sandra Strobel

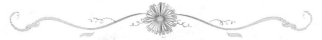

November 5

We cried together and sat in silence together—we grew close over that weekend—nursing is caring for patients and families alike.

—Cathy Bullick

November 6

Professional nursing is a constant because our care and focus remains the same: the patient.

—Randi Kowalski

November 7

He did not need a great deal of physical care, but he needed a nurse to recognize his real need and respond to it.

—Lynn Smith

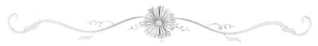

November 8

Our purpose statement (in NICU) includes not only providing a nurturing environment for optimal patient outcomes, but also being an advocate for patients and their families in all (and that is a big all) aspects of care.

—Teri O'Brien

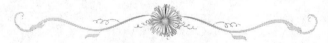

November 9

I didn't know what to do for her, so I just sat next to her. I patted her hand, stroked her arm, and just sat there with her. I felt as helpless as she did. We didn't speak; we just sat there. Later that night, this patient died. The power of presence I hope I never forget.

—Teri Vega-Stromberg

November 10

The surest test of discipline is its absence.

—Clara Barton

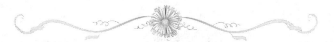

November 11

Our workplaces seldom encourage nurses to use the right sides of their brains, but doing so can strengthen our understanding of our own work and our patients' experiences.

Diana Mason (*The American Journal of Nursing,* p. 7)

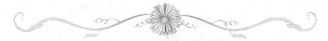

November 12

Nurses make it happen. They often save lives. At the very least, they make life a little better for the time a patient has left.

—Sharon Hudacek

November 13

Although nursing is a valued service in many social groups, it is frequently in short supply for those who need it.

—Dorthea Orem (*Nursing: Concepts of Practice*, p. 1980)

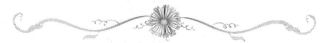

November 14

How often have you paused at the end of a particularly challenging shift and wondered, Why am I here?" I am proud to say I am a nurse. But sometimes we forget why we entered the nursing profession.

—Susan Yeakel

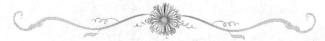

November 15

Every cold cloth applied to her forehead, every mouth swab, or every position change in bed was done with compassion and caring.

—Cathy Bullick

November 16

I love being a nurse. My mother was a nurse. I remember her coming home with stories of how she helped patients and the impact they had on her life. I knew that I wanted to be able to have that effect on someone someday.

—Meg Gambrell

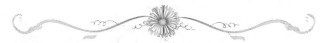

November 17

Nursing has grown as a national resource and has evolved from a procedure or activity-oriented vocation to a goal-directed professional service for health.

—Margaret Newman (*Theory Development in Nursing*, p. v)

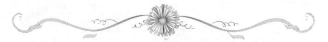

November 18

If the family cannot do it alone, it is my job as the nurse to help the patient and the family deal with this burden and this moment.

—Margaret "Peggy" Patton

November 19

It is the caring for sure, but the ordinary flow of real life cannot be discounted. The simple tasks. The genuineness.

—Sharon Hudacek

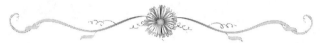

November 20

I used the skills I have been taught and adapted the nursing process to make a difference in the life of my patient and her family. I felt good.

—Anne Dolan

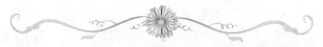

November 21

I have never been especially impressed by the heroics of people convinced that they are about to change the world. I am more awed by ... those who ... struggle to make one small difference after another.

—Ellen Goodman

November 22

Everything is not as simple as it may seem, and cookie cutter care does not apply to all. I challenge individuals to look at the whole picture; take the extra effort and be creative in her or his clinical approach.

—Susan P. Amgel

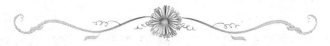

November 23

Health is the expansion of consciousness.

—Margaret Newman (*Theory Development in Nursing*, p. 19)

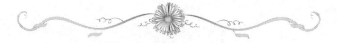

November 24

When and why people can be helped through nursing, as distinguished from other forms of human service, is a critical question for nursing.

—Dorthea Orem (*Nursing: Concepts of Practice*)

November 25

An institution or reform movement that is not selfish must originate in the recognition of some evil that is adding to the sum of human suffering, or diminishing the sum of happiness.

—Clara Barton

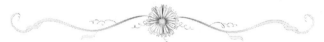

November 26

There is something that happens when two strangers participate in petitioning for divine power in one person's behalf. Suddenly, they are not strangers but two friends, asking God to help bring comfort where anxiety and pain once were.

—Allison Ash Malnar (*The Healers Art*, p. 30)

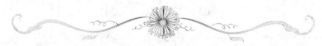

November 27

Much of Rheba's success can be attributed to her ability to build relationships and her ability to remain focused on the principal outcome of all healthcare providers—the patient.

—Beth P. Houser on Rheba de Tornyay (*Pivotal Moments in Nursing*, p. 202)

November 28

Not everything is at it seems initially,and sometimes people need a lot of encouragement.

—Charles Kemp

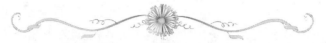

November 29

I believe that I have made my patients' lives better in many ways, but they too have made me a better person and a better nurse. It is as though I have taken a few steps in another's shoes and have gained a great deal of understanding that I would never have received otherwise.

—Nancy Hartley

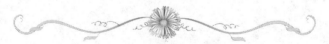

November 30

We never know when we will have to become patient advocates to help another human being, even a total stranger.

—William T. Campbell

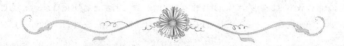

This is the finest measure of thanksgiving: a thankfulness that springs from love.

—William C. Skeath

December

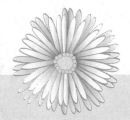

December is a time of year for peace and tranquility; it's for giving and appreciating. It's a time to prepare our hearts for self-lessness and appreciation. The December words are reflections from nurses who are inspired by the spirit of the season in comforting those from the moment life begins to the moment life ends.

The greatest gift you can have is the capacity to light your own fire.
—Henry David Thoreau

December 1

I shed more than one tear for a Christmas card I will not receive this year. You see the Christmas card will not come because my patient died around this time last year from cancer. One would think that as a nurse death might be something that is easy to cope with. I think the hardest thing is the loss of the special spirit of patients we have cared for.

—Dana Olive

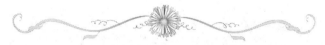

December 2

The only lights in the room were the candles in the windows and the lights from the tree. A lifetime of memories was shared as their mother (and wife) peacefully died. They were all so frightened, yet my presence gave them strength. By the time I left, several hours later, I knew I had helped this family in a very special way. Although I never knew the patient, her husband and children allowed me to share a very personal and private time with them. I entered a stranger, and left a friend.

—Sharon Quintavalle

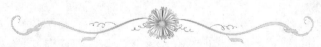

December 3

I have found in life one must be visible in fighting for what one is passionate about, and hope the rest will follow.

—Claire Fagin (*Pivotal Moments in Nursing*, p. 205)

December 4

Mary MacGregor

Mary MacGregor,
You proudly sit before me
At age 95 years
Kyphotic, curled forward
As if in anticipation
Or submission.
Your lap cradles ten gnarled fingers
That have kneaded many a loaf of bread
And have tied far too many a child's shoe.
There is a tight determined pout to your mouth.
Your face is wrinkled from the wear of laughter
And of reality.
I imagine the once young you
That tenderly embraced a young lover.
You now sit, gazing into the distance.
I know by history that you are blind.
I love the thick brogue of your native Ireland
And I know by experience not to challenge your personality.
You are here today
With a hope.
I am the guest who will share with the audience
A holistic nursing modality.
And again, you sit.
And I observe in awe and with humility
That you are waiting for me,
That you trust me.
I embrace you
With my hands
To gentle you
In that Therapeutic Touch way.
You and I, the elder and the younger
Dance a wonderful dance
Of surrender and of giving;
An exchange at soul level.
We are in the moment.
All is understood.
And, it is during times such as this
That I am truly aware
Of who the privileged one is.
For this, I am thankful.

—Mary Majkut

December 5

We are nurses, people who care. ... It may be as simple as a smile, as long as a lunch break, or a deed unnoticed. We may never know what each act of kindness does for others. As our lives pass theirs, it is always wise to reach out. "Be careful when you entertain strangers, for, in so doing, you might just entertain angels, unaware."

—Sandra Strobel

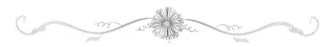

December 6

I am looking at a picture of me at Christmas at five years of age in my little nurse's uniform and reflect years later on my 30 years of nursing. I also reflect on how many patients have touched my life as well as how many patients' lives I have touched. Most of my nursing experience, almost 23 years, has been in labor and delivery—that is a lot of mothers and babies.

—Judith Sorg

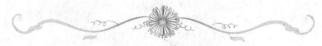

December 7

Linda is a risk taker who thrives on being told something is impossible. She is gifted in making the impossible look ordinary. She has taken the perspective of nursing to some of the most influential health care forums in the world because she is a nurse first.

—Beth P. Houser on Linda Aiken (*Pivotal Moments in Nursing*, p. 226)

December 8

After ten years, and many experiences, memories about life and death have been the most profound of all. Although I do not fully understand why, I believe that God has a purpose in everything, and allows things to happen for a reason. Patients come into your life for a reason, and God entrusts them in your care. Now, I know why I am a nurse.

—Julie A. Louder

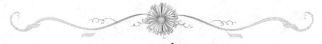

December 9

Twenty six years later ... I still shed tears and grieve.

—Teri Vega-Stromberg

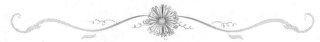

December 10

A visitor approached the nursing station like any other able body would—on two good legs. To my surprise, this was the same young man who once lived moment-to-moment, hoping to have a pain-free day. He was actually walking! It was good to realize that his goals were met and my care plan was complete, three years later.

—April Barbara Furey Reuther

December 11

Free yourself from the chains of judgment and welcome the freedom of compassion. Forgive yourself and forgive all others. Co-create tomorrow in a different fashion.

—Bonnie Wesorick (*The Way of Respect in the Work Place*, p. 42)

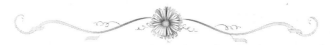

December 12

One day I cared for a woman in terrible pain. After maximum pain medication did not have enough relief, I felt frustrated. It dawned on me to give my patient a massage, a form of therapeutic touch. At first, I think she became more tense, but within ten minutes her breaths became slow and deep and her body relaxed significantly. After 20 minutes, she was asleep. She rested peacefully for about two hours.

—Katie Johnson

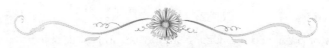

December 13

A patient is more than just a broken arm, or fluid-filled lung that needs fixing. The cornerstone of caring evolves not only around the illness, but around the patient's entire well being—physical, mental, and spiritual. Often it means taking a little extra time to show you care.

Jeffrey R. Murray

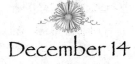

December 14

Supplicants

Not so silent supplications
Midnight prayers from bedside breaths.

Take his pain, make it mine
Bring her peace, I will struggle.
Swap our bodies, rest our souls.

Missives hurled towards heaven's ears.
Does anyone hear?

—Joanne Calore Turco (The HeART of Nursing, p. 80)

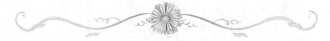

December 15

Joan never really gave up her dream of being a teacher. She is a teacher to everyone she meets. Joan just happens to be a teacher with RN after her name.

Jackie L. Sallade (*Ordinary People, Extraordinary Lives*, p. 29)

December 16

Nurses spend a lot of time trying to heal the physical body. Too often, we have preconceived notions of patients that limit our ability to care for the entire patient.

—Carolina Jensen (*The Healers Art*, p. 35)

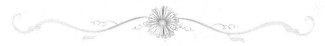

December 17

A nurse's role as an advocate and comforter has the power to transform a patient's surgical experience. Not only are patients reassured by touch, but also by a soft voice that speaks words of comfort.

—Jennifer W. Allen

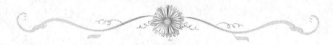

December 18

Judi knows that she has been blessed. She has a career that blends the best of all worlds—caring for patients, caring for students, and constantly being on the cutting edge of new knowledge and technology. The people who actually have been blessed are the people who have been touched by Judi.

—Vicky Keough (*Ordinary People, Extraordinary Lives*, p. 31)

December 19

Sister Joanna was truly a pioneer in the Wild West. She taught nursing staff at the bedside, she focused on providing care to the poor, she used fund raising as a way to raise money for the poor and build hospitals, and she developed an employer pre-payment system as a type of insurance for workers who might become injured or sick.

—Carolyn Hope Smeltzer and Sister Judith Jackson (*Ordinary People, Extraordinary Lives*, p. 34)

December 20

Knowledge of both nursing science and nursing art is needed for excellence in practice. ... Without language or discussion, nurses have no tools to name or claim nurse-sensitive outcomes of artful care. There is no legitimacy without language, no power without words, no answers without penetrating questions and debate.

—Kathryn Loise Gramling (The HeART of Nursing, pp. 3-4)

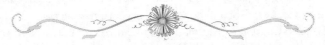

December 21

They go the extra mile. They give with their hearts, and lead with great minds.

—Sharon Hudacek

December 22

Despite breaking a rule or two at the hospital, I still know it was the best decision I ever made.

—Name withheld by request

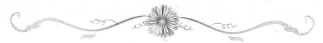

December 23

Nursing is a profession of constant giving of self in order to receive the optimal outcome: a healthy patient or individual.

—Carla Glaus

December 24

Christmas was approaching, and one special patient needed his own Christmas party, with all the trimmings. His diet was quite limited, so the cake would be targeted to please him and his cardiologist. I made an egg-beater, low-sodium, low-fat cake and decorated it like a white package with a big red ribbon. The cake, as an intervention, communicated our caring, our understanding of this man in his culture and current life situation. His eyes absolutely lit up and shined as hope. I know his last days were spent in a joyful, hopeful spirit—as a real human being, of worth and with no fear in his eyes.

—Name withheld by request

December 25

The nurses buy warm Christmas socks around the holidays for the infants in our care. One common denominator among all the infants—from the preemies on up—is the sigh of contentment that comes after their warm Christmas socks are on, and they are content and comforted.

—Mary M. Hale

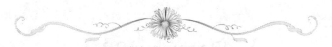

December 26

My patients give me more than they'll ever know. It is a privilege to do what I do—my memories never let me forget.

—Teresa M. Conte

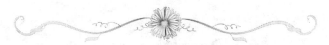

December 27

More often than not your efforts are small ones spread over many patients, and you never know which ones were successful.

—Name withheld by request

December 28

Although partially eclipsed by present day values and priorities, it is certain that nurses around the world continue to offer themselves in knowledgeable and compassionate care to those in need.

—Sharon Hudacek

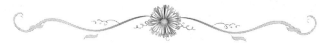

December 29

There is no better satisfaction in nursing than to witness a child transform from painful misery to peaceful respite.

—Patti Lucarelli

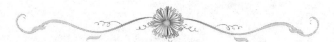

December 30

In the end, then, nursing art lies within relationships and continues to emerge because of its intense power to contribute to healing. This healing can be of the nurse, or of the patient, or of family members; it can also be healing of the profession. … For many nurses, like myself, nursing art unfolding within the crushingly vulnerable moments of clinical care can help to define the essence of nursing for us all.

—M. Cecilia Wendler (*The HeART of Nursing*, p. 116)

December 31

Their gifts are many; skillful hands, powerful intuition, gutsy advocacy.
Through it all, they are heroes, who won't take no for an answer.

—Sharon Hudacek

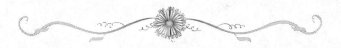

Kindness is a language which the deaf can hear and the blind can read.

-Mark Twain

References

Abrams, S. E. (1999). Saving our stories. Public Health Nursing, 16 (2), 77-78.

Benner, P. (2000). The wisdom of our practice. The American Journal of Nursing, 100 (10), 99-105.

Benner, P. (1984). From novice to expert. Excellence and power in clinical nursing practice. The American Journal of Nursing, 82(3):402-7.

Benner, P. & Wrubel, J. (1989). The primacy of caring. Stress and coping in health and illness. CA: Addison-Wesley.

Benson, E.R. (2001). As we see ourselves: Jewish women in nursing. Indianapolis, IN: Sigma Theta Tau International.

Carey, Mariah. (1993). "Hero" from the album Music Box, copyright Copyright held by The Island Def Jam Music Group/Universal Music.

Houser, B. & Player, K. (2004). Pivotal moments in nursing: Leaders who changed the path of a profession. Indianapolis, IN: Sigma Theta Tau International.

Hudacek, S. (2000). Making a difference: Stories from the point of care. Indianapolis, IN: Sigma Theta Tau International.

Leight, S. B. (2002). Starry night: using story to inform aesthetic knowing in women's health nursing. Journal of Advanced Nursing, 37 (1), 108-114.

Mason, D. (2000). Word for word. AJN, 100 (7), 7.

Muff, J. (1982). Socialization, sexism, and stereotyping. Women's issues in nursing. Illinois: Waveland.

Newman, M. (1979). Theory development in nursing. Philadelphia: F.A. Davis

Orem, D. (1980). Nursing: Concepts of practice, 2nd edition. New York: McGraw Hill.

Parker, R. S. (1990). Nurses' stories: the search for a relational ethic of care. Advances in Nursing Science, 13 (1), 31-40.

Robinson, T.M. & Perry, P.M. (2001). Cadet Nurse Stories: The call for and response of women during World War II. Indianapolis, IN: Sigma Theta Tau International.

Sandelowski, M. (1991). Telling stories: Narrative approaches in qualitative research. Image, Journal of Nursing Scholarship, 23 (3), 161-166.

Smeltzer, C. & Vlasses, F. (2003). Ordinary people, extraordinary lives: The stories of nurses. Indianapolis, IN: Sigma Theta Tau International.

Wendler, C. (2002). The heart of nursing: Expressions of creative art in nursing. Indianapolis, IN: Sigma Theta Tau International.

Wesorick, B. (1999). The way of authenticity in the work place. Grandville, MI: Grandville Printing Company.

Wesorick, B. (1999). The way of respect in the work place. Grandville, MI: Grandville Printing Company.

The Healers Art. 50th Anniversary Celebration. (2002) Brigham Young University College of Nursing. Stories collected by A.E. Bond, B. Madleco & M.L. Warnick

Contributors

Books Published by the Honor Society of Nursing, Sigma Theta Tau International

A Daybook for Nurses: Making a Difference Each Day, Hudacek, 2004.

The Adventurous Years: Leaders in Action 1973-1999, Henderson, 1998.

As We See Ourselves: Jewish Women in Nursing, Benson, 2001.

Building and Managing a Career in Nursing: Strategies for Advancing Your Career, Miller, 2003.

Cadet Nurse Stories: The Call for and Response of Women During World War II, Perry and Robinson, 2001.

Collaboration for the Promotion of Nursing, Briggs, Merk, and Mitchell, 2003.

Creating Responsive Solutions to Healthcare Change, McCullough, 2001.

Gerontological Nursing Issues for the 21st Century, Gueldner and Poon, 1999.

The HeART of Nursing: Expressions of Creative Art in Nursing, Wendler, 2002.

The Image Editors: Mind, Spirit, and Voice, Hamilton, 1997.

Immigrant Women and Their Health: An Olive Paper, Ibrahim Meleis, Lipson, Muecke and Smith, 1998.

The Language of Nursing Theory and Metatheory, King and Fawcett, 1997.

Making a Difference: Stories from the Point of Care, Hudacek, 2000.

Making a Difference: Stories from the Point of Care, Volume 2, Hudacek, 2004.

The Neuman Systems Model and Nursing Education: Teaching Strategies and Outcomes, Lowry, 1998.

Nurses' Moral Practice: Investing and Discounting Self, Kelly, 2000.

Nursing and Philanthropy: An Energizing Metaphor for the 21st Century, McBride, 2000.

Ordinary People, Extraordinary Lives: The Stories of Nurses, Smeltzer and Vlasses, 2003.

Pivotal Moments in Nursing Leaders Who Changed the Path of a Profession, Houser and Player, 2004.

The Roy Adaptation Model-Based Research: 25 Years of Contributions to Nursing Science, Boston Based Adaptation Research in Nursing Society, 1999.

Stories of Family Caregiving: Reconsideration of Theory, Literature, and Life, Poirier and Ayres, 2002.

Virginia Avenel Henderson: Signature for Nursing, Hermann, 1997.

For more information and to order these books from the Honor Society of Nursing, Sigma Theta Tau International, visit the society's Web site at www.nursingsociety.org/publications , or go to www.nursingknowledge.org/stti/books, the Web site of Nursing Knowledge International, the honor society's sales and distribution division, or call 1.888.NKI.4.YOU (U.S. and Canada) or +1.317.634.8171 (Outside U.S. and Canada).